# Techniques and Innovation in Hernia Surgery

*Edited by Angelo Guttadauro*

Published in London, United Kingdom

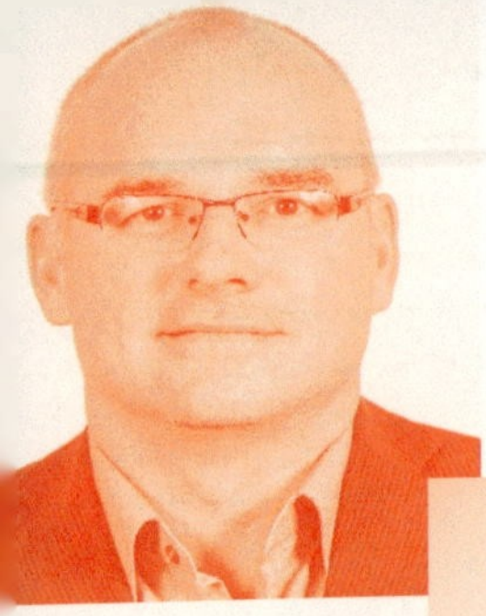
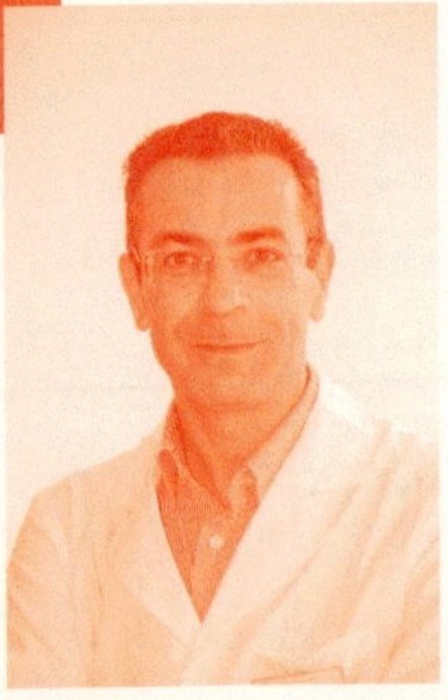
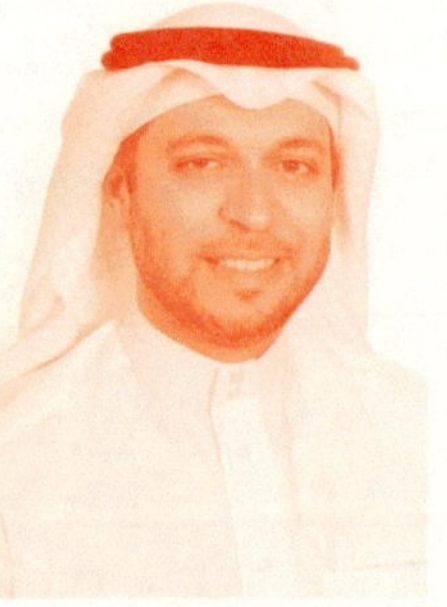
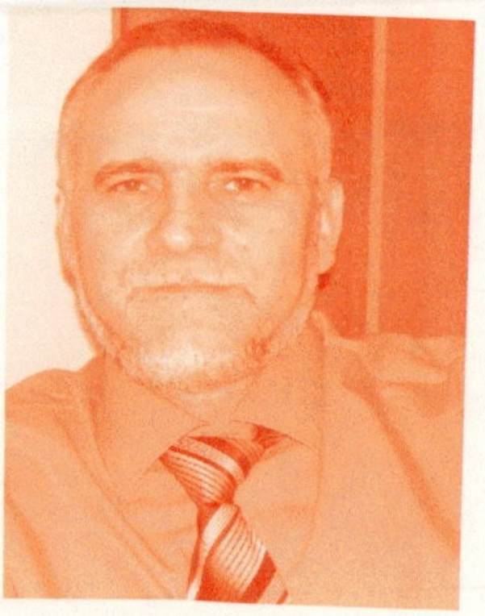
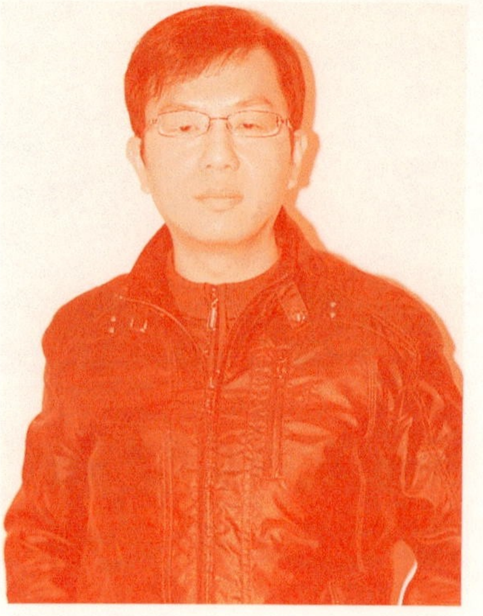
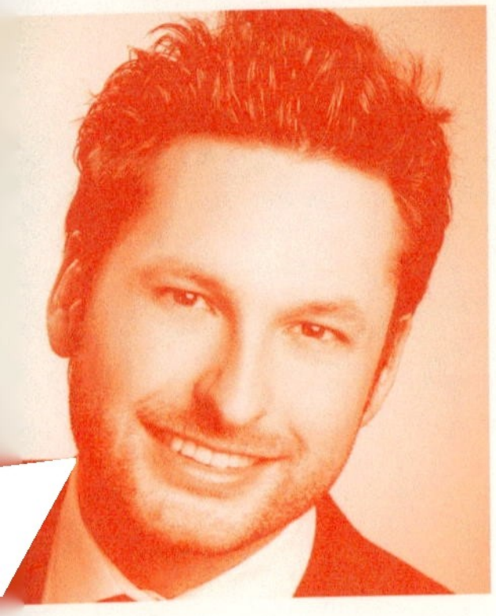
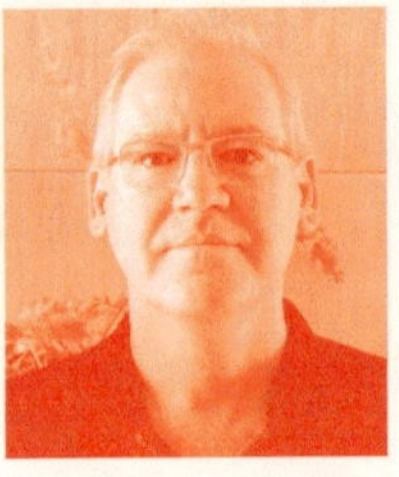

IntechOpen

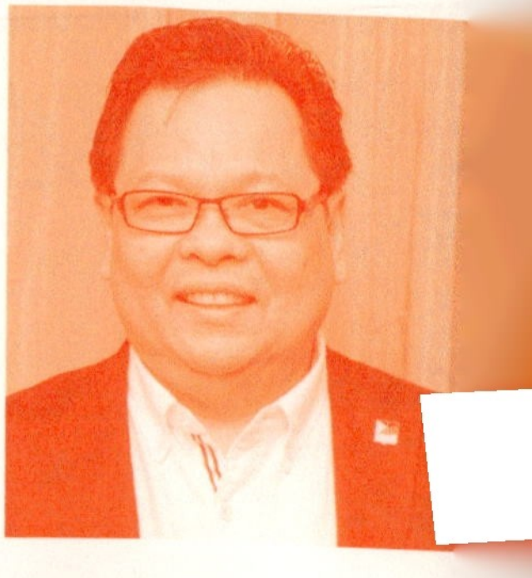
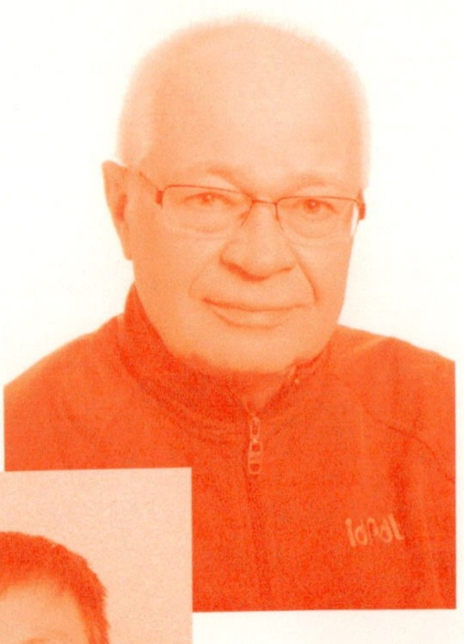
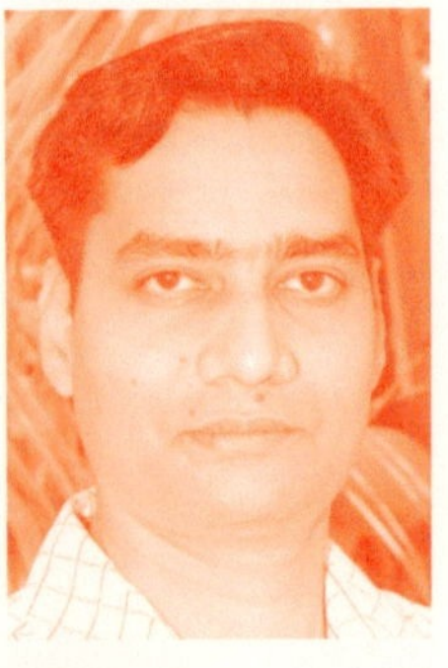
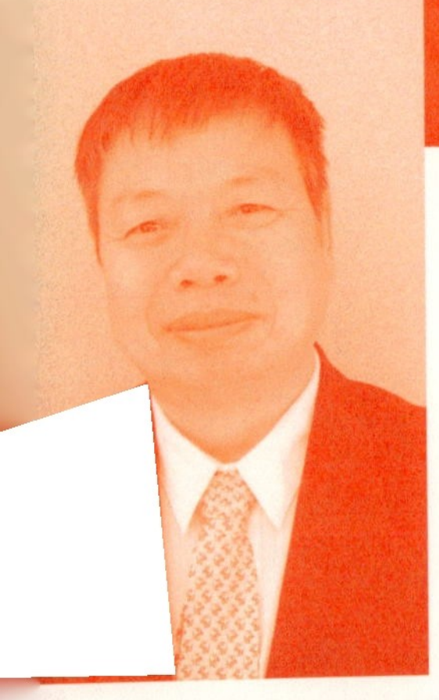
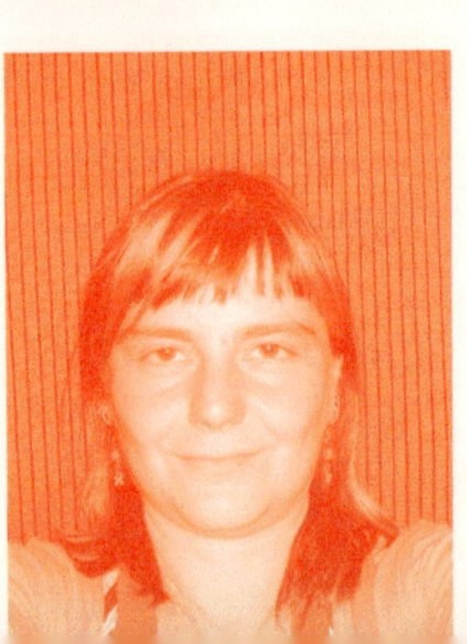
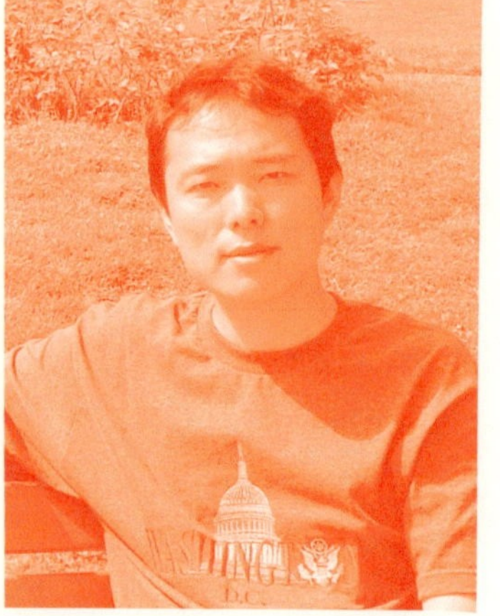

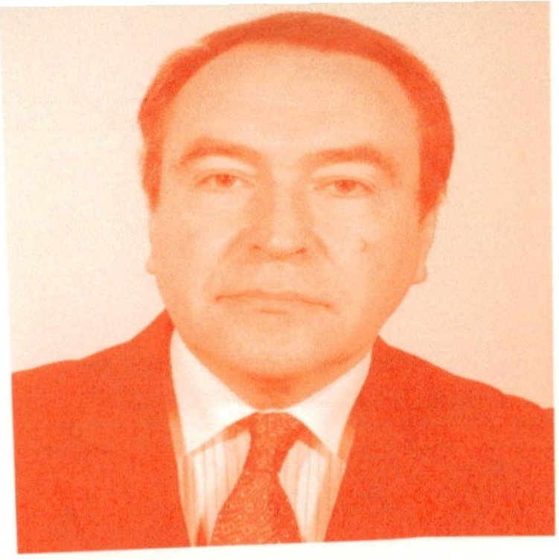
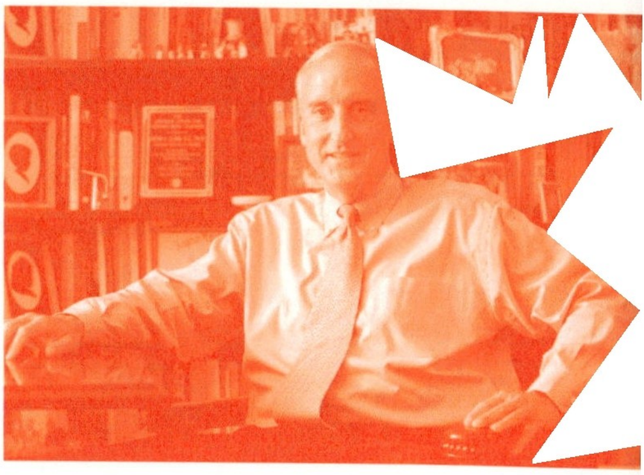
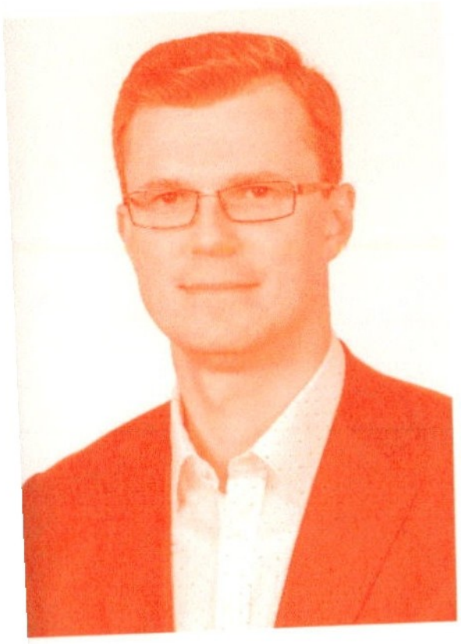
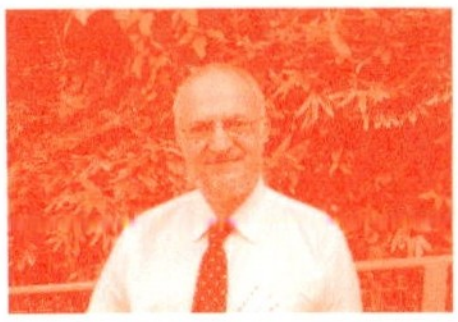
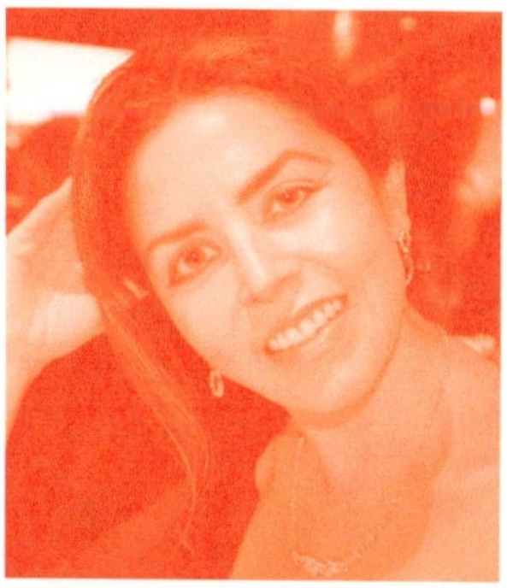

*Supporting open minds since 2005*

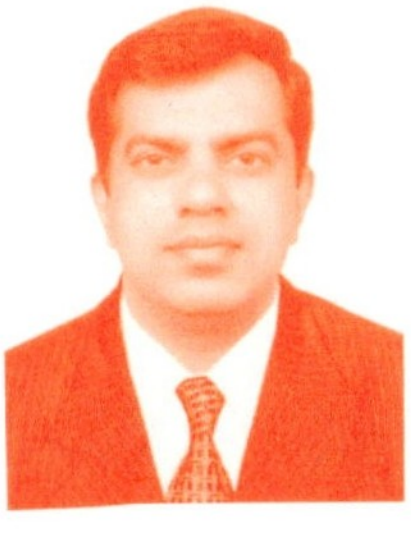
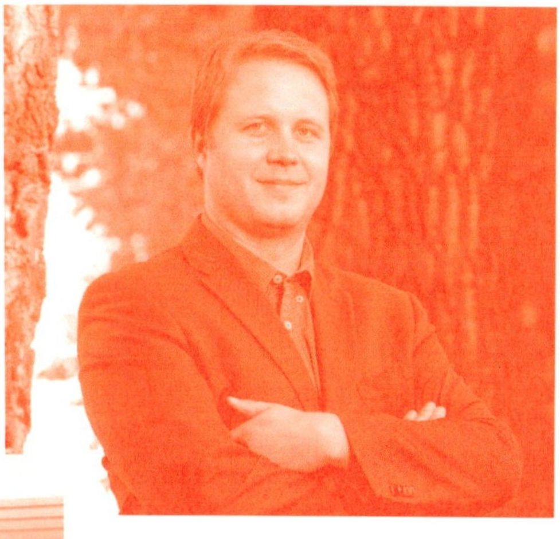
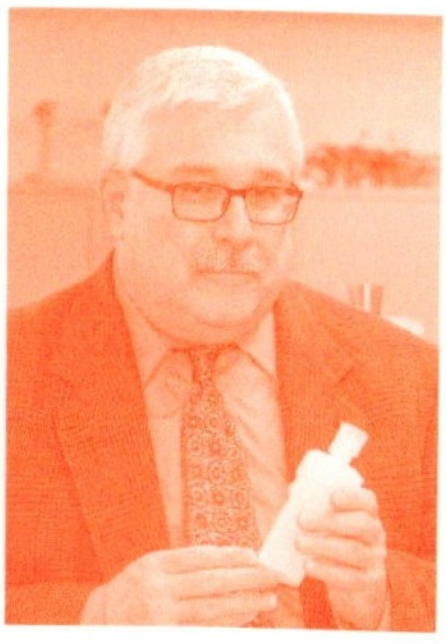
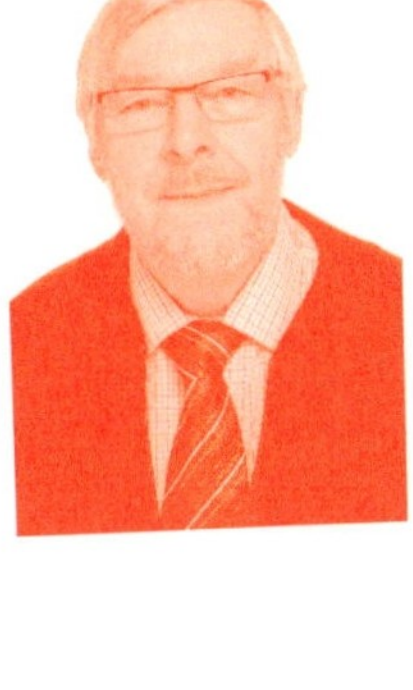
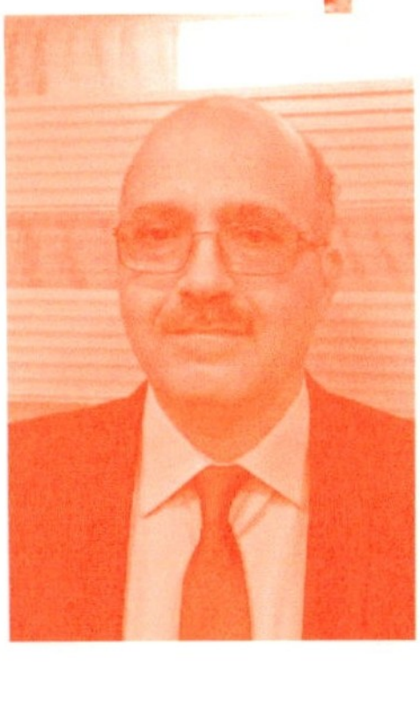
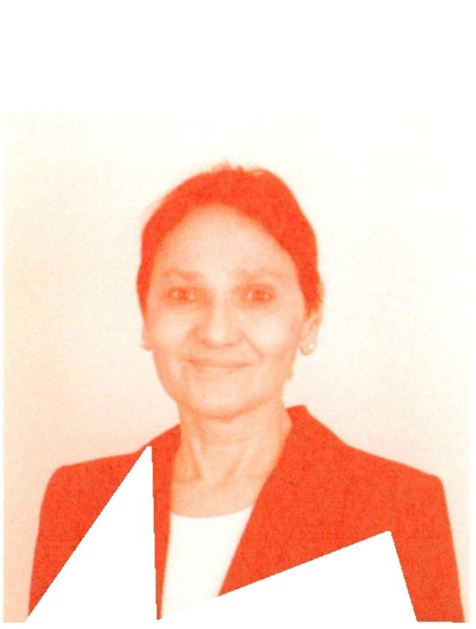
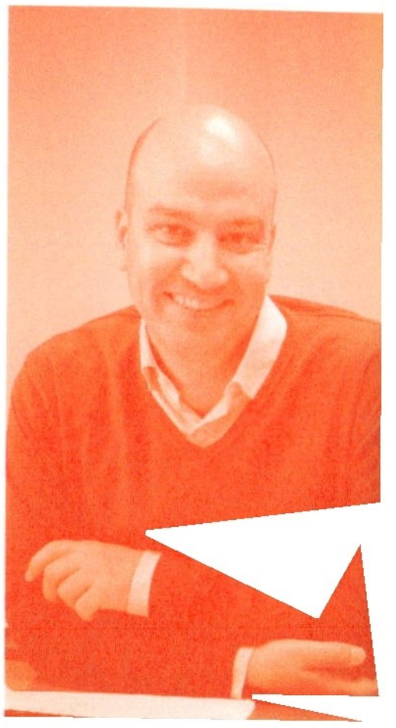

Techniques and Innovation in Hernia Surgery
http://dx.doi.org/10.5772/intechopen.83109
Edited by Angelo Guttadauro

Contributors
Abdul Mannan Khan Rao, Charles Butler, Sahil Kapur, Ashanga Yatawatta, Victor Gheorghe Radu, Anil Kumar, Shiv Paswan, Emrah Akin, Fatih Altintoprak, Reno Rudiman, Andika Winata, Frederica Jessie Tchoungui Ritz, Marco Chiarelli, Morena Burati, Angelo Guttadauro



First published in London, United Kingdom, 2020 by IntechOpen
IntechOpen is the global imprint of INTECHOPEN LIMITED, registered in England and Wales, registration number: 11086078, 7th floor, 10 Lower Thames Street, London, EC3R 6AF, United Kingdom
Printed in Croatia

British Library Cataloguing-in-Publication Data
A catalogue record for this book is available from the British Library

Additional hard and PDF copies can be obtained from orders@intechopen.com

Techniques and Innovation in Hernia Surgery
Edited by Angelo Guttadauro
p. cm.
Print ISBN 978-1-83880-147-2
Online ISBN 978-1-83880-148-9
eBook (PDF) ISBN 978-1-78985-856-3

For EU product safety concerns:
IN TECH d.o.o., Prolaz Marije Krucifikse Kozulić 3, 51000 Rijeka, Croatia, info@intechopen.com or visit our website at intechopen.com.

# Meet the editor

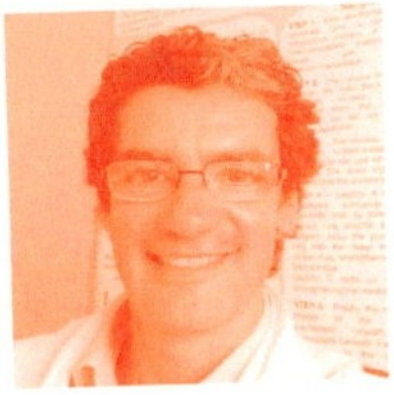

Dr Angelo Guttadauro is a researcher at the University of Milan-Bicocca and first level manager at the U.O.C. of General Surgery at the Zucchi Clinical Institutes of Monza. He is the founder and head of the "Hernia Center" of Monza-Brianza. He has participated in research projects of the Ministry of University and Scientific and Technological Research. In 2015 he obtained an international patent for a prosthesis for inguinal hernioplasty and standardized a new surgical technique for the application of the aforementioned method. In 2017 he won the Innovation Grant award of the University of Milan-Bicocca. He is the author of 78 scientific publications, books and abstracts published in national and international journals and book chapters. He has presented his works at around 200 national and international congresses.

# Contents

# Foreword

The history of medicine emphasizes that because of epidemiological relevance, the hernia has always drawn the careful attention of general practitioners and especially of surgeons. Hernia sites are many and the disease can become disabling and, with its complications, dangerous.

The surgeon's goal is to carry out an operation with fast recovery, as painless as possible. and without recurrence risk. At the end of the last century, technical improvements (especially the employment of synthetic meshes and, for certain types of hernias and laparoceles, the laparoscopic approach) led to a fundamental evolution of this surgery with a increased development of new methods of repair.

For this reason, any scientific contribution, including the various clinical aspects, is interesting, such as the evolution of new operative techniques or the evaluation of the results of methods commonly used in daily surgical activity. Recently, particular interest has been aroused by the prevention and treatment of complications and by the new problems connected with the widespread use of prosthetic materials.

This book's Editor is Dr Angelo Guttadauro, my excellent university assistant and my dear friend. Keen on this surgery even with original ideas, Dr Guttadauro has produced a good update with the contribution of specialists from several countries. The final result is effective, so I am sure that this further scientific contribution will be welcomed by all the surgeons and in particular by the specialists dealing routinely with this pathology.

**Francesco Gabrielli**
Full Professor of General Surgery,
Department of Medicine and Surgery,
University of Milano-Bicocca,
Milan, Italy

# Preface

Hernias of the abdominal wall include all cases in which the intestine protrudes from the site where it is contained due to a muscle-aponeurotic weakness or a pathological enlargement of natural orifices. Due to congenital causes and physiological ageing of the organism, all conditions of increased pressure inside the abdomen contribute to the onset of the disease.

Hernias of the abdominal wall are amongst the most treated diseases in all hospitals of the world.

Over the past 20 years, the introduction of prostheses in hernia surgery has almost completely replaced plastic abdominal wall interventions that use the patient's tissues to repair the hernial defect. Almost simultaneously, the introduction of laparoscopy has contributed to innovation in the treatment of this disease.

Today there are hundreds of types of non-absorbable, partially or fully absorbable, biological synthetic prostheses. New surgical techniques, conformed to the introduction of new types and forms of prosthetic material, can guide the surgeon in choosing the best approach for each individual patient.

Many interventions that treat hernial disease can now be performed in most parts of the world in outpatient surgery with local anaesthesia, guaranteeing a rapid recovery for the patients and an early return to normal daily activities. This has allowed for a reduction in public health spending and a greater availability of beds for the hospitalisation of more serious diseases.

Complications, however rare, seem to be minor in the centres dedicated to the treatment of hernial pathology.

The purpose of this book is to gather the experiences of distinguished authors from all over the world in order to assess the most common techniques, clarify ideas with the aim of providing guidance, and become acquainted with the most modern technological innovations.

**Dr. Angelo Guttadauro**
Researcher in General Surgery,
Department of Medicine and Surgery,
University of Milano-Biccocca,
Head of Hernia Center Monza-Brianza,
Clinical Unit of General Surgery,
Italy

Section 1

# Introduction

Chapter 1

# Introductory Chapter: State of the Art in Hernia Surgery

*Angelo Guttadauro*

## 1. Introduction

After the introduction of prostheses, wall surgery has undergone a progressive evolution aiming both at the development of new techniques and at the study of new and more comfortable prosthetic materials. Until recently the repair of a wall defect was carried out by direct suture of the muscle-aponeurotic structures and related to a high incidence of recurrence and postoperative pain. With the use of prostheses, surgeons are now able to adopt techniques and technologies more respectful of the original anatomy and physiology, avoiding tension between the muscle and tendon structures. This allows to reduce drastically the incidence of recurrence. Laparoscopy and robotic surgery, when used with the correct indications, are less traumatic and invasive and reduce postoperative pain. The higher costs allegated to these procedures are, in some cases, at least partially mitigated by the patient's better postoperative course and to a more rapid resumption of his work.

## 2. Tailored surgery

Today there are numerous open and laparoscopic surgical techniques available for the treatment of the various types of wall defects. The choice of the most appropriate technique for a specific patient remains fundamental. The concept of "tailored surgery" is new in this field and is based on the fact that each type of hernia and each patient are different from the other. Therefore surgical procedures should not be chosen according to the normal protocols but based on the needs and characteristics of that specific patient such as age, physical constitution, life habits, and work activity, but above all the size and type of the hernia should be considered. This would allow an effective treatment with the best comfort for the patient, minimal hospitalization, and most rapid resumption of normal activities.

## 3. Problems

Among abdominal wall hernias, inguinal hernia repair is the most frequently performed surgical operation in all operating rooms around the world. Since the 1970s, one of the priorities in inguinal hernia surgery was that of minimizing postoperative chronic pain [1, 2]. All surgical techniques proposed during the few past years to improve patient's comfort reported a variable incidence of neuralgia [1–4] that, when persistent after 3–6 months from surgery, may compromise significantly the patient's quality of life. Pain may be related to the presence of the mesh that, depending on its size and location, may take contact with muscular structures or cause fibrotic entrapment of nerves when in subfascial position [5–7]. Studies



IntechOpen

conducted on animals also showed perineural alterations with myelinic degeneration due to contact between nervous structures and the mesh [8], hence the necessity of identifying and dissecting subfascial nerves [9] and even of dividing them to avoid chronic pain [9, 10]. This led to the setting of guidelines for the prevention and treatment of chronic neurotic pain following inguinal hernioplasty [11, 12].

The all-in-one mesh hernioplasty technique [13], proposed by myself a few years ago, is a procedure that employs a smaller precut single mesh that covers all weak areas of the inguinal canal and is enveloped in the fibro-cremasteric sheath, avoiding the contact of the prosthesis with neural structures. Because of its shape, the mesh is placed in a deeper site directly over the weak areas of the floor of the inguinal channel, and, although smaller, it doesn't seem to increase the rate of recurrence. The more common Lichtenstein technique provides that the prosthesis is laid on the transversalis fascia and fixed to the sides becoming necessarily underaponeurotic in the upper third. In our technique, the prosthesis is positioned and remains on the transversalis fascia being covered with the fibro-cremasteric sheath. The mesh is anchored to the inguinal floor by a single point at the pubic tubercle and comprises a section that is introduced inside the deep inguinal ring. Therefore the mesh is not directly underaponeurotic at any level, stays in place, and therefore does not require lateral fixation. In addition, the prosthesis is not in contact with the ilioinguinal and iliohypogastric nerves. This new procedure may have technical advantages and help less experienced surgeon to avoid pitfalls in dealing with nerves. According to our series, "all-in-one mesh" hernioplasty presents a low rate of long-term complications. Employing a smaller amount of prosthetic material, placed where no contact with nerves occurs, avoids neuralgia and sensation of foreign body.

## 4. Conclusion

The task of a good surgeon today is to know how to choose, based on your experience and taking into account innovation. The best technique correctly tailored on the patient guarantees the best results.


## Author details

Angelo Guttadauro[1,2]

1 Department of Medicine and Surgery, University of Milan-Bicocca, Italy

2 Hernia Center Monza-Brianza, Clinical Unit of General Surgery, Zucchi Clinical Institutes of Monza, Italy

*Address all correspondence to: angelo.guttadauro@unimib.it

## References

[1] Pierides GA, Paajanen HE, Vironen JA. Factors predicting chronic pain after open mesh based inguinal hernia repair: A prospective cohort study. International Journal of Surgery. 2016;**29**:165-170

[2] Campanelli G, Sfeclan C, Cavalli M, et al. Reducing postoperative pain: The use of Tisseel for mesh fixation in inguinal hernia repair. Surgical Technology International. 2012;**22**:134-139

[3] Kehlet H, Roumen RM, Reinpold W, et al. Invited commentary: Persistent pain after inguinal hernia repair: What do we know and what do we need to know? Hernia. 2013;**17**:293-297

[4] Bueno J, Serralta A, Planells M, et al. Inguinodynia after two inguinal herniorrhaphy methods. Surgical Laparoscopy Endoscopy & Percutaneous Techniques. 2004;**14**: 210-214

[5] Fischer JE. Hernia repair: Why do we continue to perform mesh repair in the face of the human toll of inguinodynia? The American Journal of Surgery. Oct 2013;**206**(4):619-623

[6] Karakayali F, Karatas M, Ozcelik U, et al. Influence of synthetic mesh on ilioinguinal nerve motor conduction and chronic groin pain after inguinal herniorrhaphy: A prospective randomized clinical study. International Surgery. 2007;**92**:344-350

[7] Heise CP, Starling JR. Mesh inguinodynia: A new clinical syndrome after inguinal herniorrhaphy? Journal of the American College of Surgeons. 1998;**187**:514-518

[8] Demirer S, Kepenekci I, Evirgen O, et al. The effect of polypropylene mesh on ilioinguinal nerve in open mesh repair of groin hernia. Journal of Surgical Research. 2006;**131**:175-181

[9] Alfieri S, Rotondi F, Di Miceli D, et al. Chronic pain after inguinal hernia mesh repair: Possible role of surgical manipulation of the inguinal nerves. A prospective multicentre study of 973 cases. Chirurgia Italiana. 2006;**58**:23-31

[10] Mui WL, Ng CS, Fung TM, et al. Prophylactic ilioinguinal neurectomy in open inguinal hernia repair: A double-blind randomized controlled trial. Annals of Surgery. 2006;**244**:27-33

[11] Alfieri S, Amid PK, Campanelli G, et al. International guidelines for prevention and management of post-operative chronic pain following inguinal hernia surgery. Hernia. 2011;**15**: 239-249

[12] Graham DS, MacQueen IT, Chen DC. Inguinal neuroanatomy: Implications for prevention of chronic postinguinal hernia pain. International Journal of Abdominal Wall and Hernia Surgery. 2018;**1**(1):1-8

[13] Guttadauro A, Maternini M, Frassani S, De Simone M, Chiarelli M, Macchini D, et al. "All-in-one mesh" hernioplasty: A new procedure for primary inguinal hernia open repair. Asian Journal of Surgery. 2018;**41**(5):473-479. DOI: 10.1016/j.asjsur.2017.07.003

Section 2

# Ventral Hernia

Chapter 2

# Ventral Hernia: Causes and Management

*Abdul Mannan Khan Rao*

## Abstract

Ventral hernia is the most common type of hernia after inguinal hernias. The term "ventral hernia" creates some confusion, because in most countries of the world, especially in Europe, it is considered as incisional hernia, while in the USA, it is usually considered as hernias of anterior abdominal wall except groin hernias. Daily in the world millions of abdominal surgeries are being performed by both open or conventional and laparoscopic techniques, with 3–20% incidence of incisional. That's why mainly incisional hernia and its causes, risk factors, and predisposing conditions and management will be discussed in this chapter, though other ventral hernias will be described briefly. The important causes, risk factors [congenital and acquired (patients and postoperative)], and predisposing conditions for ventral hernias will be discussed in detail. The signs and symptoms produced by ventral hernia (incision) will be described initially and later, and how to investigate to confirm the diagnosis and necessary investigations before surgery for different types of patients is described. In managing the ventral hernia, different treatment options are discussed and described, like conservative management, open method, laparoscopic technique, and more advanced robotic technique. After surgery postoperative care of patient and wound is also discussed.

**Keywords:** hernia, ventral, incisional, anterior abdominal wall defect, open technique, laparoscopic technique

## 1. Introduction

In general term, the ventral hernia is the protrusion of intra-abdominal contents, through the anterior abdominal wall fascia defect [1], except groin hernia. In this way ventral hernia may be umbilical, paraumbilical, epigastric, incisional, Spigelian, parastomal, and lumbar. Sometimes this term creates confusion, because in Europe the term "ventral hernia" is used for incisional hernia, while in USA, this term is used for abdominal wall hernia, other than groin hernias [2]. In this chapter we will focus more on incisional hernias because worldwide this is a more common surgical problem.

Primary abdominal hernia can occur spontaneously at any area of natural weakness of abdominal fascia and muscles. Unlike abdominal wall hernias, which occur through a weak anatomical point, incisional hernias occur through a weakness at the site of abdominal wall closure after surgery. Ventral (incision) hernia is a common complication after open abdominal surgeries with an incidence of approximately 10% [3]. The true incidence is difficult to determine; the reasons for this are the lack of standardized definition, the inconsistency of data sources, and short length of follow-up. The reported incidence of incisional hernia after midline laparotomy is 3–20% and becomes doubled if the wound gets an infection [4]. Usually 50% of incisional hernias are detected within 1 year of surgery, but they can occur several years after surgery, with a subsequent risk of 2% per year [5].

Every year in the world, millions of abdominal surgeries are performed for different indications, and incisional hernia is one of the major complications of these surgeries, resulting in an increased morbidity and putting burden of cost on patients. It is estimated that each year approximately 10,000 repairs are performed in the UK, and 100,000 are performed in the USA [6].

Ventral hernias occur through anteriolateral abdominal wall; the structure of this wall consists of many layers including the skin, fat, fascia, muscles, and peritoneum. The order of abdominal wall layers change at different location. Above the arcuate line (imaginary line between the umbilicus and pubic symphysis), the fascia of internal oblique aponeurosis envelopes the rectus sheath. The external oblique aponeurosis always lays anterior to the internal oblique aponeurosis and the transversus abdominis aponeurosis always posterior to it. Below the arcuate line, all three layers of aponeurosis become anterior to the rectus muscle, and it is no longer enveloped. The only fascial layer below the rectus is the transversalis fascia which is separated from the transversus abdominis aponeurosis [7, 8]. These layers work together to give strength to the abdominal wall and prevent the intestine, omentum, and other tissues from bulging out.

## 2. Causes and risk factors

Causes of ventral hernia may be congenital (Ehlers-Danlos syndrome, Marfan's syndrome, etc.) or acquired (surgery, trauma). If patient developed abdominal hernia having no previous surgery at the hernia site, these are often due to weakness in the abdominal wall present at birth. As the patient becomes older or injured, these weaknesses can worsen, leading to hernia. Other risk factors are:

- Pregnancy
- Obesity
- History of previous hernia
- History of abdominal surgeries
- Injuries to abdominal wall
- Family history of hernia
- Frequently lifting or pushing heavy objects
- Chronic cough
- Straining during defecation or micturition
- Some medicines, such as steroid

Incision hernia (ventral) can occur after any abdominal surgery, but they are more common in some patients, such as:

- Old patient
- Obese patient
- Diabetics
- Patients using steroid
- Lung disease
- Smoking
- Surgical site infection
- Postoperative repeated vomiting
- Postoperative abdominal distention (intestinal obstruction)

All these have been related to increased incisional hernia rate. This occur most often after a long incision in the middle of the abdomen, but they can occur through incisions anywhere on the abdomen [9]. Sometimes these hernias developed only in part of the incision.

After abdominal surgery, if persistent or repeated, intra-abdominal pressure increased from any cause (ileus, ascites, etc.) can lead to microscopic tears of scar. Over time this can decrease the strength of tissue, predisposing patient to develop hernia. Tissue strength following surgery can only achieve an 80% tensile strength of previous healthy tissue; this is an additional effect in the formation of incisional hernia. In this way after second midline laparotomy, the maximum tissue strength would be 80% of 80%, which will be 64%, and this 80% predicted tensile strength in under perfect conditions, assuming no evidence of malnutrition or wound infection. If these conditions are present, the chance of incisional hernia formation further increases.

Until now it is thought that incisional hernia results mainly from a technical failure in the surgical closure of the abdominal wall. However it is known that, there are complex patients, surgical and post operative, variables influence incisional hernia development.

## 3. Patient factors

Patients with some connective tissue diseases (Marfan's syndrome, osteogenesis imperfecta, and Ehlers-Danlos syndrome) have increased the incidence of incisional hernia [10, 11]. It is concluded from research that collagen metabolism in patients with a hernia is changed at three levels.

- The ratio between type I collagen (strong) and type III collagen (weak) is decreased.
- The quality of collagen is poor.
- Collagen breakdown is increased via increased matrix metalloproteinase (MMP) activity [12].

| Risk factors | Effect on wound healing |
|---|---|
| Old age (>65 year) | Decreased collagen formation and reduced tissue perfusion |
| Atherosclerosis | Wound blood perfusion reduced |
| Diabetes | Alteration in microcirculation and reduced inflammatory response |
| Obesity | Increased risk of wound infection, presence of obesity related comorbid diseases (diabetes, atherosclerosis, etc.) |
| Malignancy or debilitating diseases | Increase chance of malnutrition, wound infection, wound dehiscence, poor wound healing |
| Renal failure | Abnormal metabolic conditions prevent normal granulation tissue |
| Protein deficiency | Reduced collagen formation |
| Immunosuppression | Increased chance of wound infection, alteration in normal tissue regeneration |
| Smoking | Vasoconstriction and repeated increased intra-abdominal pressure from coughing |
| Drugs (steroid, etc.) | Immunosuppression, reduced vascular perfusion |
| Vitamin C deficiency | Reduced collagen formation |

**Table 1.**
*Patient-related risk factors for incisional hernia development.*

However it has not been clear and established whether these changes are localized to the hernia site or whether it affects all body tissues. Other patient-related risk factors are shown in **Table 1**.

## 4. Operative factors

Though incisional hernias can occur after any type of laparotomy incision, they are most common after midline (especially upper midline) and transverse incisions [5] .The incidence of incisional hernia after midline abdominal incision is approximately 10.5, and 7.5% after transverse incisions [9]. Research shows that a continuous closure technique with simple running sutures is the best option for closure of laparotomy incisions [13, 14]. The use of slowly absorbable monofilament suture material versus

| Risk factors | Effect on wound |
|---|---|
| Midline incisions | Result in increased incidence of incision hernia |
| Suture material | The use of slowly absorbable monofilament has a better result |
| Suture technique | Sutures having small bite reduce the incidence of incision hernia and wound infection |
| Homeostasis | Good bleeding control reduces the chance of wound infection |
| Ratio of suture length to wound length | If it is >5.1, it may result in an increased incidence of wound infection |
| Overuse of diathermy | Result in more necrotic tissue in wound; this increases the incidence of wound infection |
| Prophylactic use of mesh | Reduces the incidence of incision hernia |
| Prophylactic antibiotic | Reduces the chance of wound infection |

**Table 2.**
*Showing surgical factors that affect incidence of incision hernia.*

nonabsorbable or braided material decreases the rate of incisional hernia and reduces the postoperative wound infection [13, 14]. Suture length used with ratio to wound length between 4:1 to 5:1 minimizes the risk of incisional hernia [15, 16]. Traditionally surgeons close laparotomy wound with continuous suture placed 10 mm apart and 10 mm away from edge. Recent studies shows that large tissue bites have been shown to be associated with an increase in the amount of necrotic tissue and slackening of the stitches, resulting in increased risk of wound infection and the development of an incisional hernia [17, 18]. Small stitches placed 4–6 mm from the wound edge and 4 mm apart (in the aponeurotic layer only) minimized the risk of incisional hernia from 18 to 5.6% and reduced wound infection rates by 50% [19]. According to recent studies, the surgeon should adopt a small bite technique instead of large bite technique; it may result in better outcome. Surgical factors are summarized in **Table 2**.

## 5. Postoperative factors

The most important and common factor that results in incision hernia formation is wound infection, and it is thought to double the risk$^{1/4}$. Other factors are increase in intra-abdominal pressure in the immediate postoperative period, such as postoperative ileus, coughing, vomiting, and mechanical ventilation, and also increase in the risk of incisional hernia [20].

After laparotomy, the risk of incisional hernia cannot be eliminated except by avoiding a laparotomy incision. However the risk can be minimized by reducing systemic risk factors, especially smoking, obesity, and nutritional deficiencies, and by optimizing diabetic management. The risk can be further minimized by meticulous surgical technique; when closing the abdominal wall, homeostasis should be secured properly; diathermy use should be avoided to lessen the necrotic tissue in wound; if surgeon suspects that the wound may ooze, drain can be used, but it should be removed as early as possible, to reduce the incidence of wound infection. Prophylactic use of antibiotic at the time of anesthesia induction reduces the incidence of wound infection.

## 6. Signs and symptoms

Ventral hernia usually presents as painless bulge or lump in abdomen under the skin, which increases in size over time. Sometimes it presents as only discomfort in abdomen and sometimes discomfort or pain with bulge. Sometimes ventral hernia may cause pain when a patient:

- Cough
- Strains during defecation
- Stands or sit for long time
- Lifts or pushes heavy objects

Usually in initial stage, the hernia disappears when the patient lies down and then reappears or enlarges when a patient stands or lifts or pushes something heavy; this is reducible hernia. When the tissues or content inside the hernia becomes adherent to the sac or with each other, then the hernia becomes irreducible. When hernia content becomes stuck or trapped in abdominal muscle, it can cause pain, nausea, vomiting, constipation, etc. If the hernia content especially intestine gets tightly trapped in the

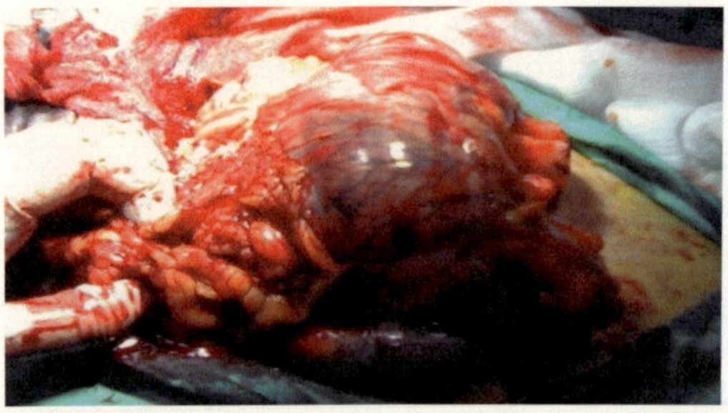

**Figure 1.**
*Gangrenous bowel of patient in **Figure 2** having strangulated hernia.*

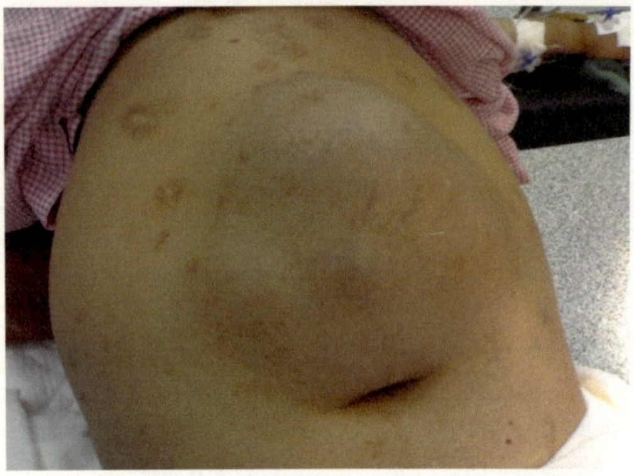

**Figure 2.**
*Strangulated ventral hernia and content are shown in **Figure 1**.*

tear in the muscles, layer or intestine loop is constricted at the narrow neck of hernia sac or apex of loop of intestine adherent to hernial sac especially at fundus and becomes twisted; the blood supply to the intestine can become cut off or reduced, resulting in bowel necrosis or rupture; this may lead to a potentially life-threatening condition known as "strangulation." This condition requires emergency surgery. Other symptoms of strangulated hernia include severe abdominal pain, abdominal distention, severe nausea and vomiting, profuse sweating, increased pulse rate, and fever. Initially pain is colicky in nature; if strangulation is not relieved, it will change in character and become continuous or disappear; this is an ominous sign that the intestine becomes necrosed or dead. **Figure 1** shows necrosed/gangrenous bowel in strangulated ventral hernia.

## 7. Diagnosis and evaluation

Usually ventral hernia can be diagnosed by history and clinical examination only. If there is confusion in diagnosis or hernia is complex and complicated, one can advise ultrasound, CT scan or MRI scan, to make the diagnosis confirm and elaborate the anatomy of hernia (**Figure 3**).

Patients usually present ventral hernia as reducible swelling in abdomen or at the site or near the incision scar of previous surgery; it disappears when the patient lies down and enlarges when the patient stands, coughs, or defecates. On clinical examination, expansile cough impulse will be present. In some cases when a hernia is incarcerated or strangulated, the swelling may be erythematous. Obesity can limit the examination; it is important that the patient should be examined in a different position, as hernia can change with exertion or standing. If incision in there

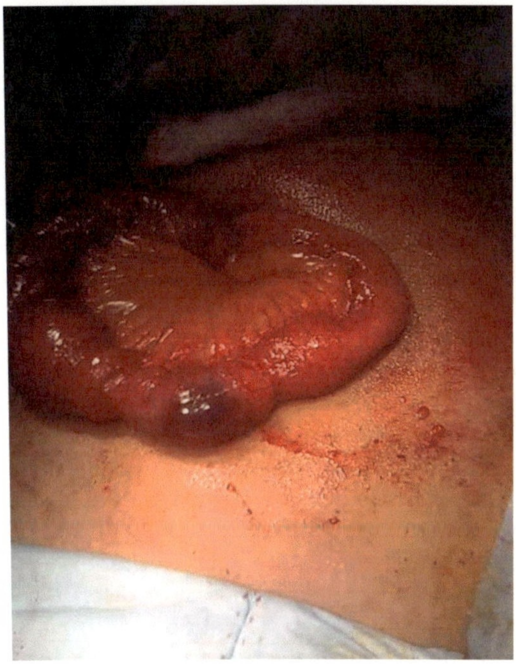

**Figure 3.**
*Showing portion of small bowel that is stuck at narrow neck of hernia.*

it should be palpated in whole length, because sometimes incisional hernia form at multiple site in a incision, and try to palpate the neck of hernia(whole in fascia at the site of incision), whether it is narrow or broad, narrow neck more prone to strangulate. Sometimes size of fascial defect may be difficult to discern clinically. The size of the peritoneal sac and associated contents is often large, although the fascial defect may be small, particularly in obese patients and after multiple abdominal operations, where there may be many small fascial defects. Usually incisional hernias are asymptomatic, but 20–50% present with pain. Skin changes may present in large and longstanding hernias.

Ultrasonography is commonly used to confirm the clinical diagnosis. The ultrasonography in hernia can reveal the fascial gap with protruding hernia contents. The hernia should increase in size or change location when the patient coughs. Bowels are characterized by peristaltic movement and inside air, whereas the omentum appears as a stationary, space-occupying structure.

In some patients of ventral hernia, detailed diagnostic imaging (ultrasonography, CT scan, and MRI) is indicated; these are:

- Obese patients (BMI > 35)
- Patients with recurrent incisional hernia
- Patient having huge hernia (second abdomen)
- Patients having pain within the abdominal wall but with no physical and detectable hernia.

In these patients CT scan with 3D reconstruction is useful. Occult hernia is accurately delineated; the content of sac is defined.

## 8. Management

Whenever the patient develops hernia, it will not get better on its own and can get worsen (enlarge) over time. The most common treatment of ventral hernia is surgery. Some hernias are repaired on an elective basis like asymptomatic hernia, but hernia which presents with strangulation requires immediate surgery. Irreducible or incarcerated hernia without strangulation is not a surgical emergency. The risks and benefits of surgery should be discussed with the patient. The patients with reasonable operative risks should have their hernia repaired within a sensible time frame. Nonsurgical management of ventral hernias with the use of binders, trusses, or corsets is considered to be ineffective. This may be the only option in a patient who is not a reasonable candidate for surgery [21–23].

In the past, before appropriate meshes and techniques for implanting them were available, sutures alone were used to close the weakness in the abdominal wall. These often were unsuccessful in the long term, as in most patients hernia would recur. For some very small ventral hernias, suturing alone remains acceptable.

Commonly ventral hernias are repaired by making an incision over the fascial defect in the abdominal wall. The intestine, fat, or other organs in the hernia are placed back in the abdomen. The defect in muscle or fascia is then closed with sutures alone or is reinforced with mesh. The abdominal wall is then closed with suture over the mesh. Sometime drainage tubes are placed through the skin to prevent serum or blood collection.

At present many types of surgical techniques have been developed to repair hernias. The most important tension-free repair is using mesh. If mesh is used, it should be placed 3 to 5 cm overlapping the edges of the fascial defect. Mesh should be handled meticulously to prevent surgical site infection. The most basic approach is primary open repair without mesh; this is typically reserved for defect in the fascia of less than 2 cm. Open mesh repair has several options, including what type of mesh and where to place the mesh. Main methods of ventral hernia repair are:

- Open hernia repair
- Minimally invasive hernia repair (laparoscopic)
- Robotic ventral hernia repair

Laparoscopic ventral hernia repair, when we compare it with open hernia repair, showed decreased overall complication rate, decreased hospital length of stay, and a quicker return to work. The disadvantage of laparoscopy includes a higher potential for visceral injury, and it is technically more difficult.

Robotic ventral hernia repair has also become popular secondary to increased freedom of motion during surgery. Closing the fascial defect robotically is far easier from a technical standpoint than attempting it with classical laparoscopic instruments. Robotic surgery is more expensive and has longer operative times than laparoscopy.

Not all patients of incisional hernia are suitable for surgical repair, and the risk of surgery must be balanced against the risk of complication if the hernia is left untreated. Small incisional hernia invariably enlarges with times as a result of the continuous intra-abdominal pressure, diaphragmatic contractions, and increased pressure from coughing or straining. Despite recent advances in the management of incisional hernias, the recurrence rate is still high. The method of choice for repair of incisional hernia is still debatable.

*DOI: http://dx.doi.org/10.5772/intechopen.88873*

It is found that incisional hernia repair without prosthetic mesh is associated with high recurrence rate, whereas hernia repair with mesh results in low recurrence rate. It is accepted that only the small(less than 3 cm) incisional hernia can be repaired by primary tissue approximation with sutures.

## 9. Laparoscopic repair

Worldwide surgeons use laparoscope to repair the incisional/ventral hernias with promising results. A composite or coated mesh (to reduce the bowel and visceral adhesions) is placed in the intra-peritoneal position, and the hernia is usually not closed. This is said to be an intra-peritoneal onlay mesh. The advantages of the laparoscopic approach are that it allows the whole of the previous incision to be visualized and small fascial defect can be identified, but at the same time it has the disadvantage of relying fully on the strength of the mesh and its fixation. Another disadvantage of laparoscopic repair is that it is criticized for producing cosmetically worse results than the open repair because the hernia sac is not excised and the defect is not closed. Furthermore, laparoscopic repair is not always possible for large incisional hernias or when the hernia extends towards the costal margin or pelvis because adequate mesh overlap cannot easily be achieved.

## 10. Open mesh repair

In practice there are three types of open repair for incisional hernia with mesh—the inlay, onlay, and sublay techniques.

In the inlay method, the mesh is placed between the muscles in a bridging position. Polypropylene mesh anchors to all adjacent tissues and can therefore induce extensive adhesions to the viscera if placed in position where it becomes adjacent to the bowel. The mesh can erode into the intestine and may result in entero-cutaneous fistulas. Recurrence rate for inlay technique is also high: These are the main drawbacks of this method. Therefore this technique is not recommended. Furthermore, the force needed to dislocate a bridged mesh is much lower than for a closed defect.

In the onlay method, the mesh is placed in the subcutaneous prefascial space, over the abdominal wall closure. The main criticism of this method is the high incidence of wound infection and seroma formation.

In the sublay technique, the mesh is placed over the closed posterior rectus sheath and peritoneum. In case if hernia is large and the posterior sheath cannot be closed, the mesh is sometimes used to bridge the defect (gap). The European Hernia Society has adopted a sublay mesh repair as a gold standard open repair.

Common surgical complications after ventral hernias repair are wound infection, mesh infection, seroma, hematoma, recurrence, ileus, intestinal adhesions, injury to abdominal organs, and chronic pain. If pain presents for more than 3 months postoperatively after incisional hernia repair, it is termed as chronic pain. The cause of the pain is poorly understood but probably includes a combination of mesh associated inflammation and nerve damage from mesh fixation.

## 11. Giant incisional hernia

If incisional hernia has a fascial defect more than 10 cm in transverse diameter, it can be considered as giant incisional hernia. If the patient is obese (BMI > 35), then there are more surgical and anesthetic challenges. These patients often have poor quality abdomen wall musculature; in addition there may be multiple comorbid medical problems. In giant incisional hernia, a further problem that has to be overcome is the risk of serious "loss of domain" once the hernia is repaired, which can result in an abdominal compartment syndrome. Loss of domain implies that a proportion of the abdominal contents entered in the hernia sac permanently outside the natural abdominal cavity. With time abdominal cavity become small, and after long time, if these abdominal contents again reduced to abdominal cavity in hernia repair, it will result in increase intra-abdominal pressure, which result in respiratory compromised and reduced venous drainage, and reduced abdominal organs perfusion.

In such cases to prevent this catastrophe complication, it is necessary to increase the intra-abdominal cavity space, before hernia repair, so that abdominal cavity could be able to accommodate hernia contents easily without increasing intra-abdominal pressure. Preoperative pneumoperitoneum has been used to overcome the problem of loss of domain by increasing the size of the abdominal cavity before hernia repair. Although this technique may be effective, it has not been widely adopted.

The compartment separation technique allows a flap of the rectus muscles, anterior rectus sheath, internal oblique, and transversus abdominis muscle to slide medially, enabling giant hernia defect to be closed. It can be reinforced with mesh.

## 12. Ventral hernia and pregnancy

In premenopausal women, the repair of large incisional hernia imposed especial problems, because elasticity and expansion of the abdominal wall will be needed if the patient subsequent becomes pregnant. Prosthetic mesh reduced the elasticity of abdominal wall enough to cause complication during pregnancy. Small incisional hernia can be left safely until the completion of family. If hernia is large and symptomatic, then it should be fixed, and in these cases it may be better to avoid the use of mesh and to use a sutured repair such as the shoelace technique. It is necessary to warn the patient about the high risk of recurrence with subsequent pregnancy.


## Author details

Abdul Mannan Khan Rao
College of Medicine, Qassim University, Saudi Arabia

*Address all correspondence to: mannanchohan66@hotmail.com

## References

[1] Malangoni MA, Hernias RMJ. In: Townsend et al., editors. Townsend: Sabiston Textbook of Surgery. 19th ed. New York: Saunders; 2012. pp. 1114-1140

[2] Sanders DL, Kingsnorth AN. The modern management of incisional hernia. BMJ. 2012;**344**:37-42

[3] Santora T, Roslyn J. Incisional hernia. The Surgical Clinics of North America. 1993;**73**:557-570

[4] Mudge M, Hughes LE. Incisional hernia: A ten year prospective study of incidence and attitudes. The British Journal of Surgery. 1995;**72**:70-71

[5] Bucknall TE, Cox PJ, Ellis H. Burst abdomen and incisional hernia: A prospective study of 1129 major laparotomies. BMJ. 1982;**284**:931-933

[6] Rutkow IM. Demographic and socioeconomic aspects of hernia repair in the United States in 2003. The Surgical Clinics of North America. 2003;**83**:1045-1051

[7] Aquina CT, Fleming FJ, Becerra AZ, Xu Z, Hensley BJ, Noyes K, et al. Explaining variation in ventral and inguinal hernia repair outcomes: A population-based analysis. Surgery. 2017;**162**(3):628-639

[8] Holihan JL, Alawadi ZM, Harris JW, Harvin J, Shah SK, Goodenough CJ, et al. Ventral hernia: Patient selection, treatment, and management. Current Problems in Surgery. 2016;**53**(7):307-354

[9] Carlson MA, Ludwig KA, Condon RE. Ventral hernia and other complications of 1000 midline incision. Southern Medical Journal. 1995;**88**(4):450-453

[10] Girotto JA, Malaisrie SC, Bulkely G, Manson PN. Recurrent ventral herniation in Ehlers-Danlos syndrome. Plastic and Reconstructive Surgery. 2000;**106**:1520-1526

[11] Klinge U, Binnebosel M, Mertens PR. Are collagens the culprits in the development of incisional and inguinal hernia disease? Hernia. 2006;**10**:472-477

[12] Henriksen NA, Yadete DH, Sorensen LT, Agren MS, Jorgensen LN. Connective tissue alteration in abdominal wall hernia. The British Journal of Surgery. 2011;**98**:210-219

[13] van 't Riet M, Steyerberg EW, Nellensteyn J, Bonjer HJ, Jeekel J. Meta-analysis of techniques for closure of midline abdominal incisions. The British Journal of Surgery. 2002;**89**:1350-1356

[14] Ceydeli A, Rucinski J, Wise L. Finding the best abdominal closure: An evidence-based review of the literature. Current Surgery. 2005;**62**:220-225

[15] Harlaar JJ, Deerenberg EB, van Ramshorst GH, Lont HE, van der Borst EC, Schouten WR, et al. A multicenter randomized controlled trial evaluating the effect of small stitches on the incidence of incisional hernia in midline incisions. BMC Surgery. 2011;**11**:20

[16] Cengiz Y, Blomquist P, Israelsson LA. Small tissue bites and wound strength: An experimental study. Archives of Surgery. 2001;**136**:272-275

[17] Israelsson LA, Jonsson T. Suture length to wound length ratio and healing of midline laparotomy incisions. The British Journal of Surgery. 1993;**80**:1284-1286

[18] Harlaar JJ, van Ramshorst GH, Nieuwenhuizen J, Ten Brinke JG, Hop WC, Kleinrensink GJ, et al. Small

stitches with small suture distances increase laparotomy closure strength. American Journal of Surgery. 2009;**198**:392-395

[19] Millbourn D, Cengiz Y, Israelsson LA. Effect of stitch length on wound complications after closure of midline incisions: A randomized controlled trial. Archives of Surgery. 2009;**144**:1056-1059

[20] Makela JT, Kiviniemi H, Juvonen T, Laitinen S. Factors influencing wound dehiscence after midline laparotomy. American Journal of Surgery. 1995;**170**:387-390

[21] Heniford BT. SAGES guidelines for laparoscopic ventral hernia repair. Surgical Endoscopy. 2016;**30**(8):3161-3162

[22] Souza JM, Dumanian GA. Routine use of bioprosthetic mesh is not necessary: A retrospective review of 100 consecutive cases of intra-abdominal midweight polypropylene mesh for ventral hernia repair. Surgery. 2013;**153**(3):393-399

[23] de Vries HS, Smeeing D, Lourens H, Kruyt PM, Mollen RMHG. Long-term clinical experience with laparoscopic ventral hernia repair using a ParietexTM composite mesh in severely obese and non-severe obese patients: A single center cohort study. Minimally Invasive Therapy & Allied Technologies. 2018;**11**:1-5

Chapter 3

# Laparoscopic Retromuscular Repair of Ventral Hernias: eTEP and eTEP-TAR

*Victor G. Radu*

## Abstract

Professors Jean Rives and Rene Stoppa published that the retrorectus space is the best for mesh placement in open ventral hernia repair and their technique has become the gold standard. This chapter presents a new technique in laparoscopic ventral hernia repair (LVHR), which combines the advantages of Rives-Stoppa procedure with the advantages of minimally invasive surgery (MIS)—it is about enhanced-view totally extraperitoneal (eTEP) approach. Restoration of the architecture of the abdominal wall and also of its functionality and the possibility to extend laterally the retromuscular dissection, if it is needed, performing transversus abdominis release (TAR) give laparoscopic retromuscular repair of ventral hernias the chance to become the gold standard in LVHR.

**Keywords:** eTEP, eTEP-TAR, laparoscopic ventral hernia repair, abdominal wall reconstruction, laparoscopic retromuscular repair, laparoscopic rives-Stoppa

## 1. Introduction

In 2012 Jorge Daes published the enhanced-view totally extraperitoneal (eTEP) approach in inguinal hernia repair. His procedure inspired Igor Belyansky to extend the retrorectus dissection cranially and cross over the midline, remaining outside of the peritoneal cavity and connecting both the retrorectus spaces. In this way he performed endoscopically the Rives-Stoppa procedure (eRS) and transversus abdominis release (eTEP-TAR), respectively, publishing a novel approach in ventral hernia repair.

### 1.1 History

The laparoscopic techniques in ventral hernia repair are improved from the "bridged-IPOM" performed by Leblanc in the 1990s to "IPOM plus"—a concept introduced 20 years later by J.F. Kukleta, who closed the defect and used the mesh for augmentation of the abdominal wall repaired [1, 2].

The evolution did not stop there and conversely still continues by not trying to find the ideal mesh but instead the ideal mesh placement. In 2002 Marc Miserez repaired a ventral hernia placing the mesh pre-peritoneally, and Wolfgang Reinpold placed the mesh under the rectus muscles by trans-hernial access (MILOS technique) [2–4].



IntechOpen

In 2016, Igor Belyansky published a new technique combining the eTEP access described by Jorge Daes with the principles of TAR described by Yuri Novitsky [5–8]. The result (eRives/eTEP-TAR) is very promising, and the technique has the potential to become one of the best solutions in laparoscopic ventral hernia repair (LVHR) [6].

## 2. Ventral hernia classification

In 2009, a group of international experts from EHS published a new classification of ventral hernias, based on location and dimensions of the hernial defect.

The primary ventral hernias are classified as medial (epigastric and umbilical) and lateral (spigelian and lumbar). In relation with the diameter, these hernias can be small, medium, or large (**Table 1**) [9].

In a similar way, the ventral incisional hernias can be medial or lateral.

The medial incisional hernias are located in the area limited by xiphoid (cranially), pubic symphysis (caudally), and the lateral edge of rectus muscles.

An easily memorable classification from M1 to M5 going from the xiphoid to pubic bone was proposed. Therefore, they define 5 M zones [9]:

Classification of the midline incisional hernias includes five zones, from xiphoid process to pubic symphysis from 3 to 3 cm (**Figure 1**).

- M1: subxiphoidal
- M2: epigastric
- M3: umbilical
- M4: infraumbilical
- M5: suprapubic [9]

The borders of the lateral area are defined as:

1. Cranial: the costal margin
2. Caudal: the inguinal region
3. Medial: the lateral margin of the rectal sheath
4. Lateral: the lumbar region

In this way, the lateral hernias are classified as follows (**Figure 2**).

- L1: subcostal
- L2: flank
- L3: iliac
- L4: lumbar

Measurement of the incisional hernias.

| EHS Primary Abdominal Wall Hernia Classification | | Diameter cm | Small <2cm | Medium ≥2-4cm | Large ≥4cm |
|---|---|---|---|---|---|
| Midline | Epigastric | | | | |
| | Umbilical | | | | |
| Lateral | Spigelian | | | | |
| | Lumbar | | | | |

**Table 1.**
*The European hernia society classification for primary abdominal wall hernias [9].*

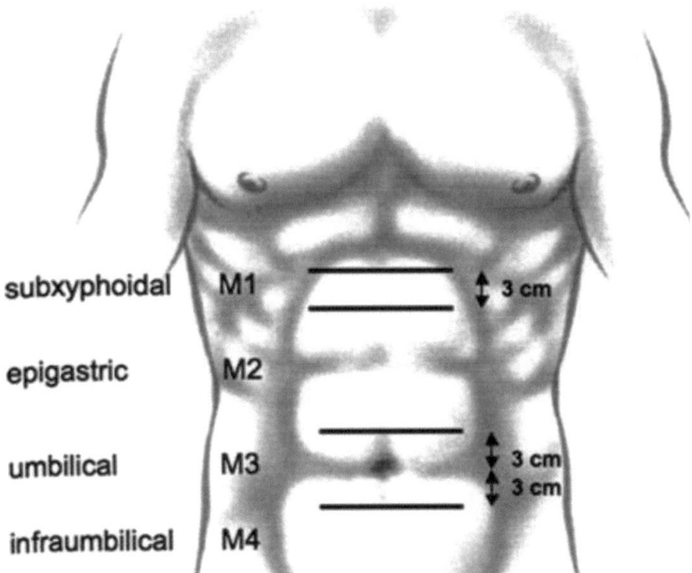


**Figure 1.**
*To classify midline incisional hernias between the two lateral margins of the rectus muscle sheaths, five zones were defined [9].*

In contrast to the primary abdominal wall hernias, incisional hernias come in many different sizes and shapes.

The length of the hernia defect was defined as the greatest vertical distance between the most cranial and the most caudal limit of the hernia defect. In case of multiple hernia defects from one incision, the length is between the cranial margin of the most cranial defect and the caudal margin of the most caudal defect (**Figure 3**).

This technique has no contraindications related to the width of the defects. As in open retromuscular surgery, the eTEP approach can be used to repair all varieties of ventral hernias, from small umbilical hernias to large and complex ventral hernias.

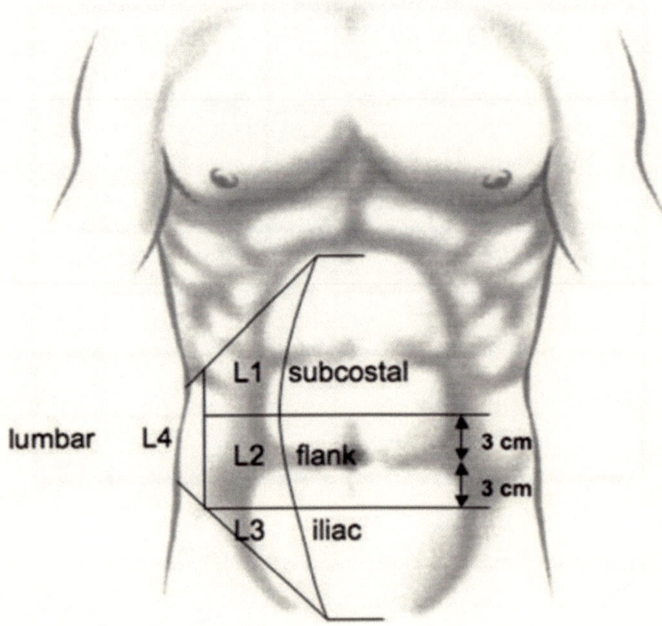


**Figure 2.**
*To classify lateral incisional hernias, four zones lateral of the rectus muscle sheaths were defined [9].*

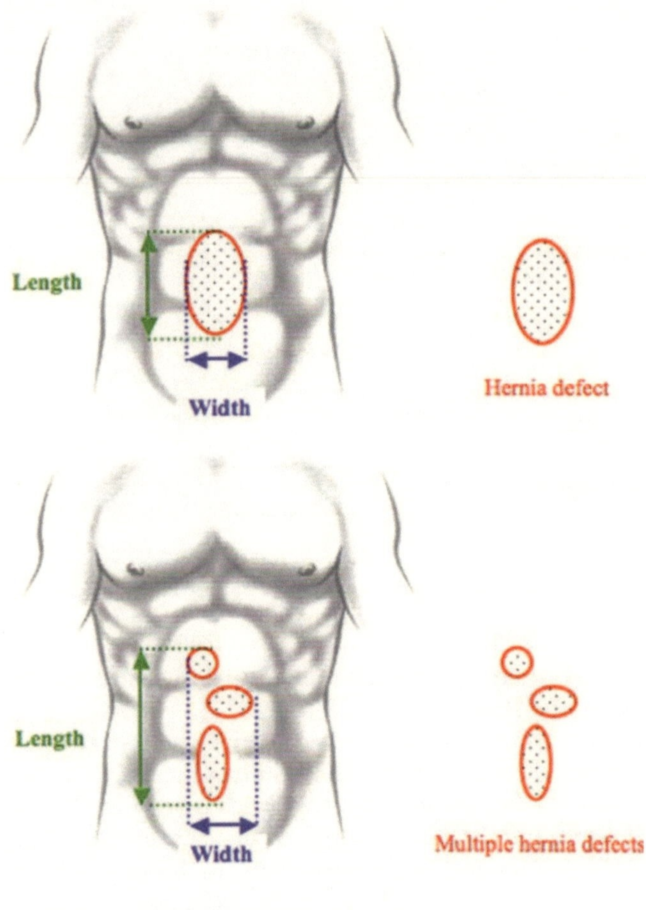


**Figure 3.**
*Definition of the width and the length of incisional hernias [9].*

## 3. The biomechanics of the abdominal wall and abdominal cavity

The advantages of the retrorectus dissection are well known. Once the rectus muscles are removed from their encasement in the rectus sheaths, linea alba can be restored, the muscles being able to be translated medially 3 cm, 5 cm, and 3 cm, respectively, in the upper, middle, and lower third of the abdomen, as Ramirez wrote in the paper describing his component separation technique. In this way large defects up to 10 cm width can be closed.

Because of an excellent arterial blood supply, the retrorectus space serves as a well-vascularized position where mesh prostheses become incorporated. This sublay mesh position has benefits at both a molecular level and a pure mechanical level. The perifilamentous collagen deposition on the mesh has a higher type I/III ratio compared with mesh placed onlay. The predominance of mature collagen (type I) confers a higher tensile strength of the wound [10].

The tone of the abdominal wall muscles induces an intra-abdominal pressure between 5 and 7 mmHg. According to Laplace's law, this pressure acts equally on the abdominal wall, determining a tension in the abdominal wall which is a positive tension (**Figure 4**) [11].

The restoration of architecture and functionality of the abdominal wall conducts restoration of the physiological tension in the abdominal wall. The focus of these procedures is the reconstruction of the linea alba, the "central tendon" of the abdominal wall.

The posterior layer will have the role of barrier between the mesh and the viscera. It is very important to suture the posterior layer totally tension free, to avoid rupture of the suture line. To suture without tension is possible preserving the peritoneal structures (the falciform ligament, the umbilical ligament, or/and the hernia sac) as a bridge between the posterior rectus sheaths. The resistance of the posterior layer will be charged by the mesh.

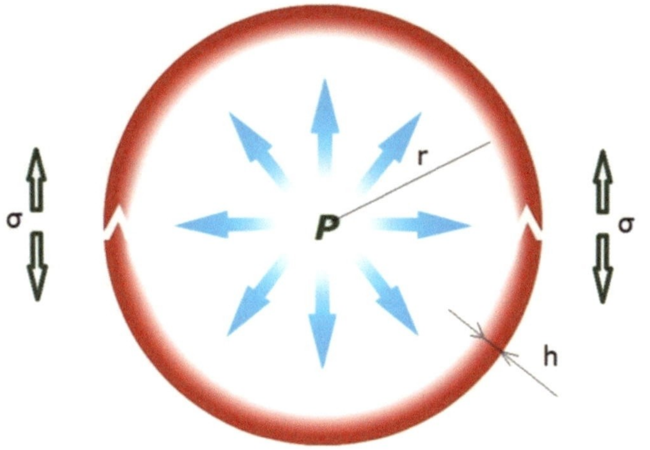


Law of Laplace: T = P x r

(T = tension; P = pressure; r = radius of cavity)

σ = T / h

(σ = stress; h = wall thickness)

**Figure 4.**
*Law of Laplace [12].*

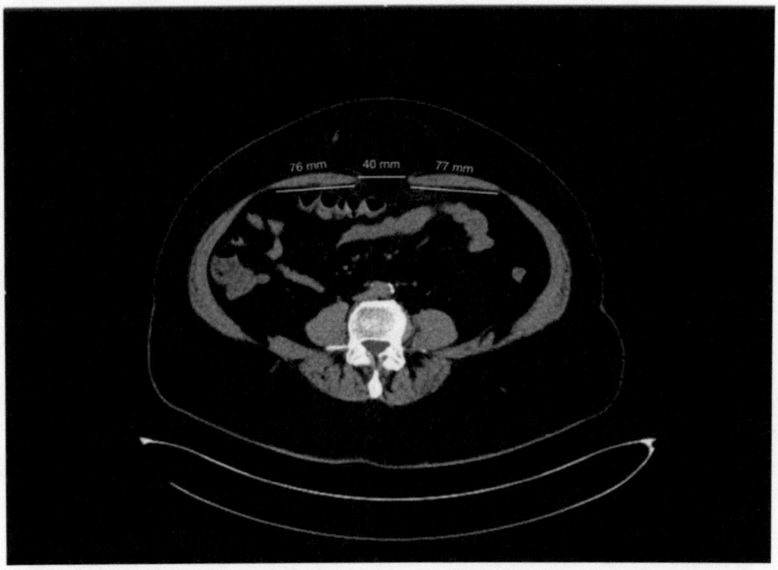


**Figure 5.**
*Carbonell's algorithm: 2xRW:DW ≥ 2:1.*

The preoperative CT scan is very useful. It allows us to locate the defect, measure it, and establish the strategy for the surgery.

Rives-Stoppa technique is sufficient when the sum of bilateral rectus muscle width is at least 2x > maximal defect width (**Figure 5**).

Additional myofascial release (TAR) may be necessary if maximal defect width closely approximates or exceeds 2x rectus width (**Figure 6**). This is Alfredo Carbonell's algorithm, presented at the 9th Annual Abdominal Wall Reconstruction Summit, Montana, USA, 2018.

The principles of the eTEP technique are:

- Closure of the defect
- Use of uncoated mesh, placed outside of the abdominal cavity
- Minimizing fixation of the mesh, without compromising the result of hernia repair

Thinking of the abdomen as a "cylinder" with many layers, the principles mentioned above can be realized, connecting three spaces:

1. The preperitoneal space, represented in the upper part of the abdomen by the falciform ligament and in the lower part of the abdomen by the umbilical ligament
2. The retrorectus spaces
3. The pretransversalis spaces, by enlarging the retromuscular dissection laterally to the semilunaris lines

Connection of these spaces can be performed crossing over the midline.

If the hernia is located in the upper part of the abdomen, crossover of the midline will be performed below the umbilicus and anterior to the umbilical ligament,

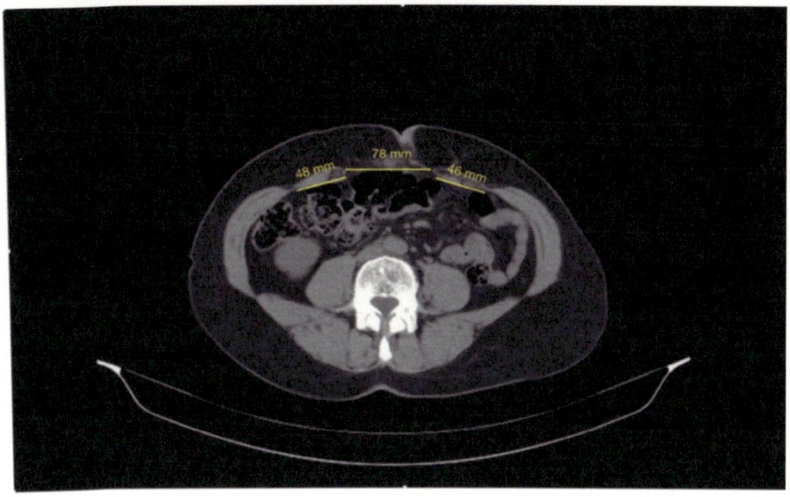


**Figure 6.**
*Carbonell's algorithm: 2xRW:DW ≤ 2:1.*

and, conversely, if the hernia is located in the lower part of the abdomen, crossover the midline will be performed from above, anterior to the falciform ligament.

The position of the patient is very important.

For the median ventral hernias, the patient will be placed in supine position, and the table will be flexed. In this position the distance between costal margins and iliac crests is increased, which allows an optimal port placement, and also the conflict is avoided between the surgeon's hand and the patient's thigh (**Figure** 7).

We will place the patient on a lateral decubitus in lateral locations of hernias, especially for lumbar hernia (L4), keeping also the table flexed. The technical aspects in repairing of lumbar hernias will be presented separately.

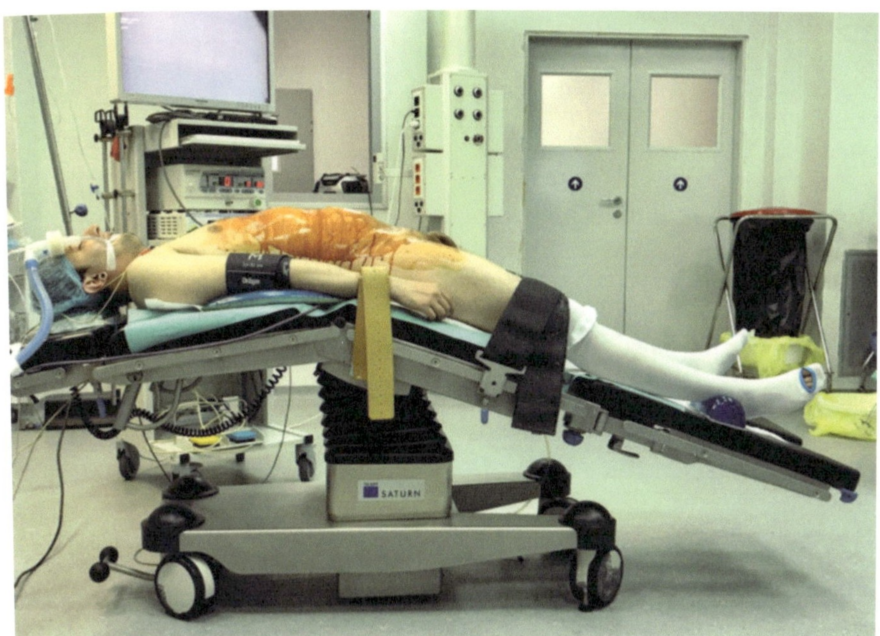


**Figure 7.**
*Position of the patient.*

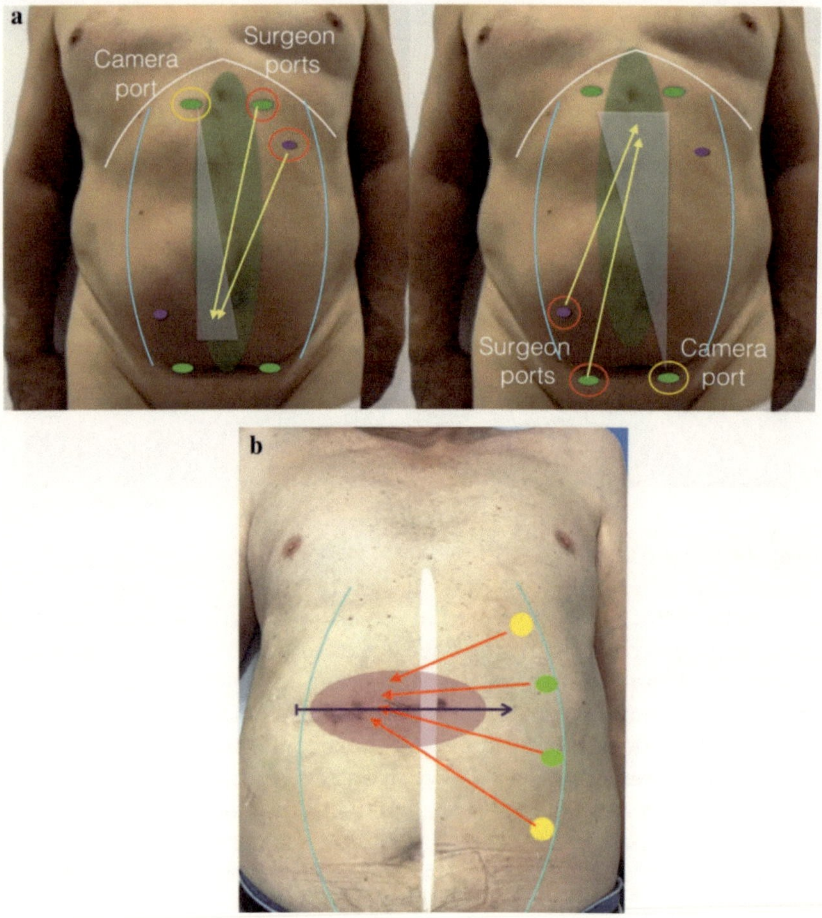


**Figure 8.**
*(a) Port placement, (b) port placement.*

The key stages of this procedure are:

1. Access of the retrorectus space and port placement

2. Crossover of the midline preperitoneally

3. Connection of both retrorectus spaces

   3* TAR (when needed [6])

4. Closure of the defect

5. Mesh placement

6. Exsufflation

1. Access of the retrorectus space and port placement.

The access of the retrorectus space is performed using an optic port placed medially to the semilunaris. The linea semilunaris is the most important landmark for port placement.

As a rule, the ports have to be placed in the opposite side of the abdomen related to the hernia location (**Figure 8a** and **b**).

After the retrorectus space is achieved by $CO_2$ insufflation, the ports are placed under direct vision just medially to the semilunaris line (**Figure 9**).

2. It is better to cross over the midline in the virgin part of the wall, on the opposite side to where the defect is located, to minimize the risk of injury of the viscera, which can be adherent to the abdominal wall.

Crossing over the midline to the contralateral retrorectus space is performed anterior to the falciform ligament, when we start from left to right (if the defect is in the lower abdomen) (**Figure 10a**) and, respectively, anterior to the umbilical ligament (if the defect is in the upper abdomen), and dissection starts from the right to left (**Figure 10b**).

3. Connection of both retrorectus spaces.

By dissection of both retrorectus spaces (left and right) and connecting them by incising the posterior sheaths on their medial aspects, we get a common large retromuscular space (the left retrorectus space connected to the right retrorectus space). This space is linked by the preperitoneal bridge represented by the falciform ligament and/or umbilical ligament. The retrorectus dissection is limited laterally by the semilunaris lines, where the neurovascular bundles pass through the posterior sheath to the rectus muscles (**Figure 11**).

3*. TAR. When the defect is too large to be closed, the TAR procedure is added. The incorporation of TAR was found beneficial in cases with a wide defect (10 cm), tension on the posterior layer, and narrow retrorectus space (< 5 cm) or when dealing with a poor compliant abdominal wall [6]. Adding the TAR is necessary for closure of the defect and also for placement of a large mesh to obtain a good overlapping.

As a right-handed surgeon, I perform TAR from the top to bottom on the right side and bottom-up on the left.

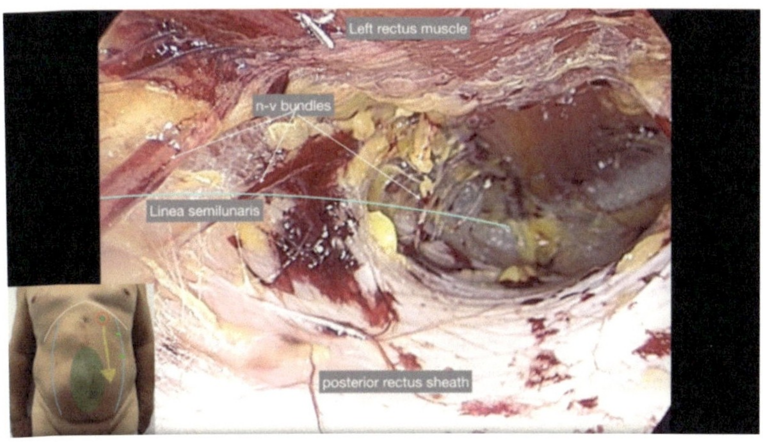


**Figure 9.**
*Development of the retrorectus space.*

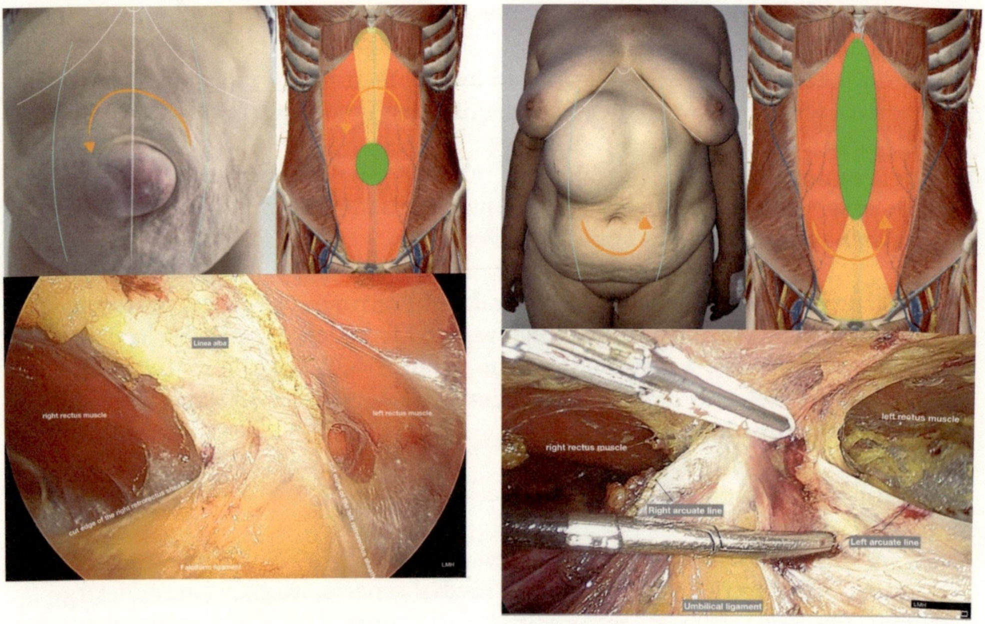


(a) (b)

**Figure 10.**
*(a) Crossing over the linea alba above the umbilicus. (b) Crossing over the linea alba below the umbilicus.*

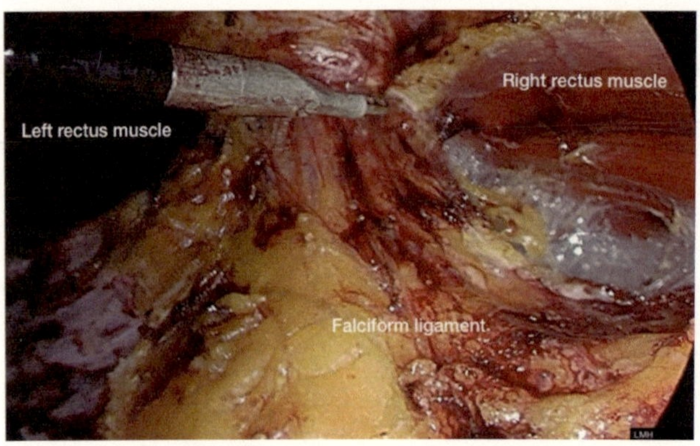


**Figure 11.**
*Retromuscular dissection: connecting both retrorectus spaces.*

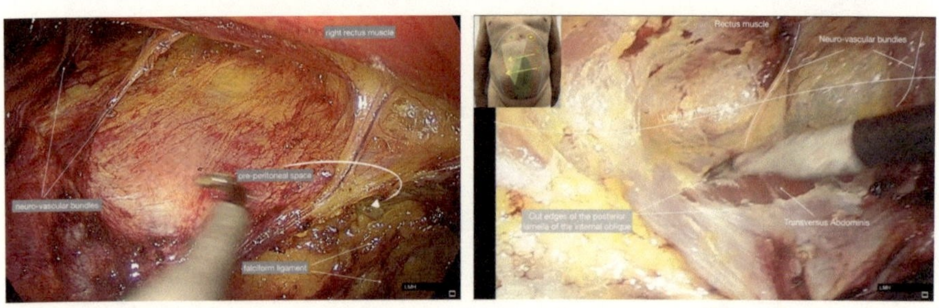


(a) (b)

**Figure 12.**
*(a) TAR top-bottom: Landmarks. (b) TAR top-bottom.*

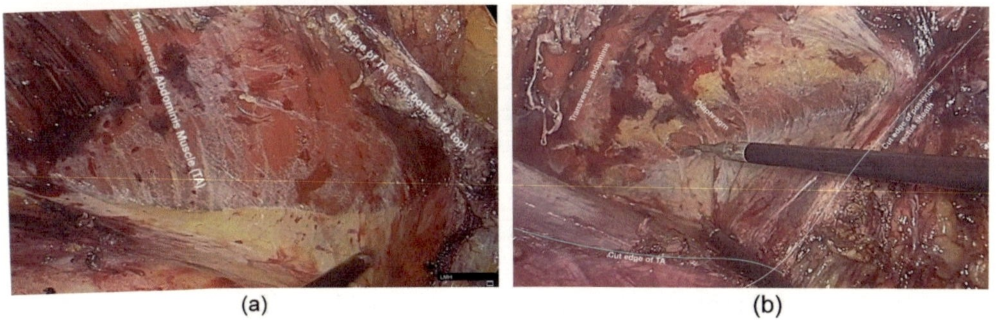


**Figure 13.**
*(a) Posterior component separation. (b) Posterior component separation.*

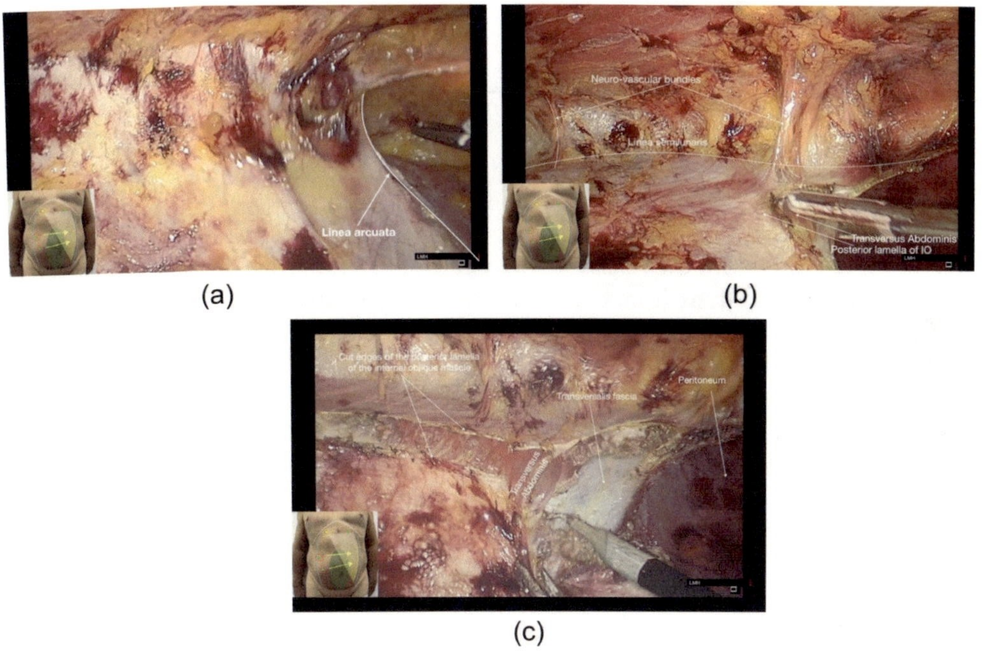


**Figure 14.**
*(a) Landmark: linea arcuata. (b) TAR bottom-up. (c) TAR after cutting of the posterior lamella of I.O.*

### 3.1 Top-bottom TAR

It is easy to identify the transversus abdominis fibers through transparency of the posterior rectus sheath. Before drawing the TAR cutline, it is necessary to see the neurovascular (NV) bundles and the semilunaris line (**Figure 12a**). The TAR line will be placed medially to these structures.

First the posterior lamella of the internal oblique muscle is incised and then transversus abdominis (TA) (**Figure 12b**). The incision must be curved medially to protect the integrity of diaphragm when the dissection is extended cranially.

After TA is released, of course dissection is extended as lateral as possible and as cranial as possible depending on hernia location (**Figure 13 a** and **b**).

### 3.2 Bottom-up TAR

In addition to the previous landmarks discussed (linea semilunaris and NV bundles) in bottom-up TAR, identification of the arcuate line is necessary (**Figure 14 a**).

First the Bogros space is dissected, and the preperitoneal dissection is enlarged cranially, behind the posterior sheath. In this way TAR can be performed without cutting the peritoneum (**Figure 14b** and **c**).

Of course, enlarging dissection laterally up to the psoas muscle allows medial mobilization of the posterior rectus sheaths.

In the subxiphoidian hernia (M1), it is very important to extend dissection behind the diaphragm. Keeping the right anatomical plane, dissection can be extended up to the central tendon of diaphragm (**Figure 15**). It is important to mention that in all the cases, there is a landmark of the limit between the transversus abdominis and diaphragm. This limit is represented by a thin fatty tissue—"the yellow line" (**Figure 16**).

In the suprapubic hernia (M5), a large retropubic prevesical dissection is recommended to obtain a good overlap.

**Some aspects to keep in mind:**

- TAR lines must be curved medially to the top to connect to subxiphoidian space and protect integrity of the diaphragm.

- The TA and diaphragm are in the same anatomical plane; they are separated by a thin fat tissue, which is very constant.

- In caudal direction, the release of TA must pass the arcuate line to get a large fascial flap, and there is no tension in the suture of the posterior layer.

4. Closure of the defect and restoration of linea alba

The defect in the posterior layer has to be closed as barrier between the mesh and the bowel (**Figure 17**).

Restoration of the linea alba is the aim of this technique. This is achieved closing the defect by suturing the anterior rectus sheaths on midline (**Figure 18**).

It is recommended to keep in the suture the peritoneal sac; in this way dead space is avoided, and postoperative seroma occurrence is prevented.

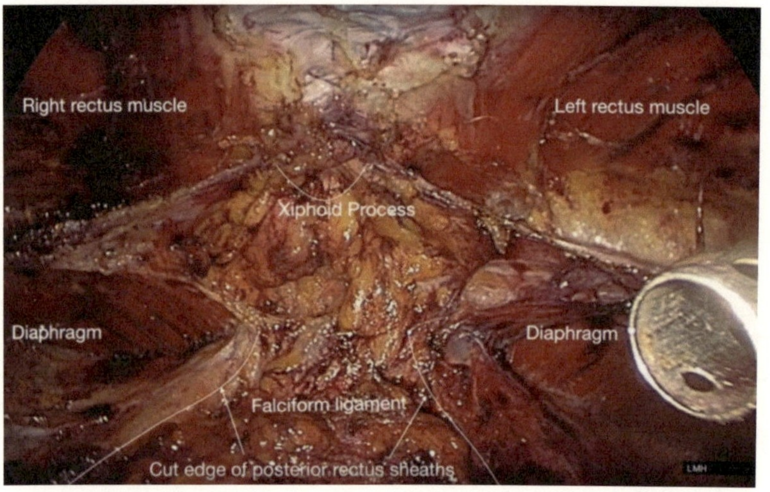


**Figure 15.**
*Dissection behind the xyphoid process.*

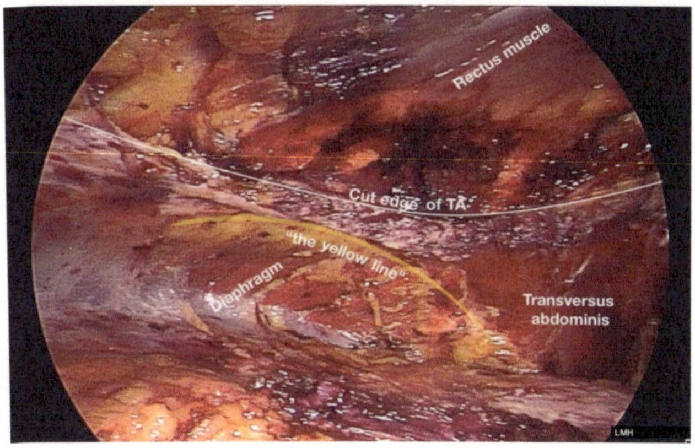


**Figure 16.**
*"Yellow line": The limit between the transversus abdominis and diaphragm.*

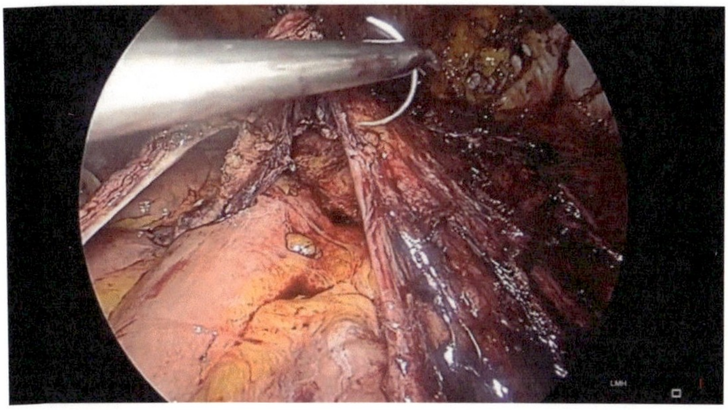


**Figure 17.**
*Closure of the posterior layer.*

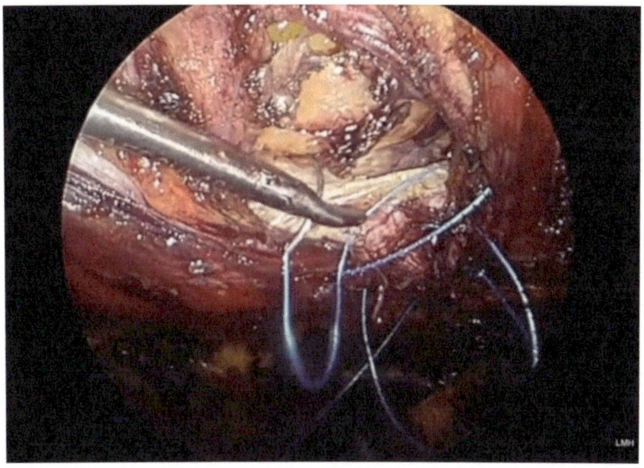


**Figure 18.**
*Restoration of linea alba.*

5. The mesh placement into the retrorectus space will be done after measurement of the entire dissected area which has to be covered by the mesh (**Figure 19**).

Usually I do not fix the mesh. A large dissection and a good overlapping, even posterior to the bones (pubic bones or costal margin) added to a correct closure of the defect, is enough for mesh fixation.

In our practice, after correct dissection and thorough hemostasis, we do not consider drainage necessary.

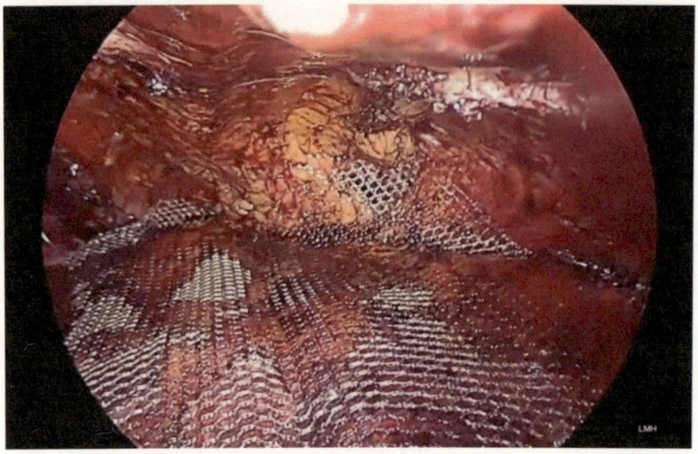

**Figure 19.**
*Mesh placement.*

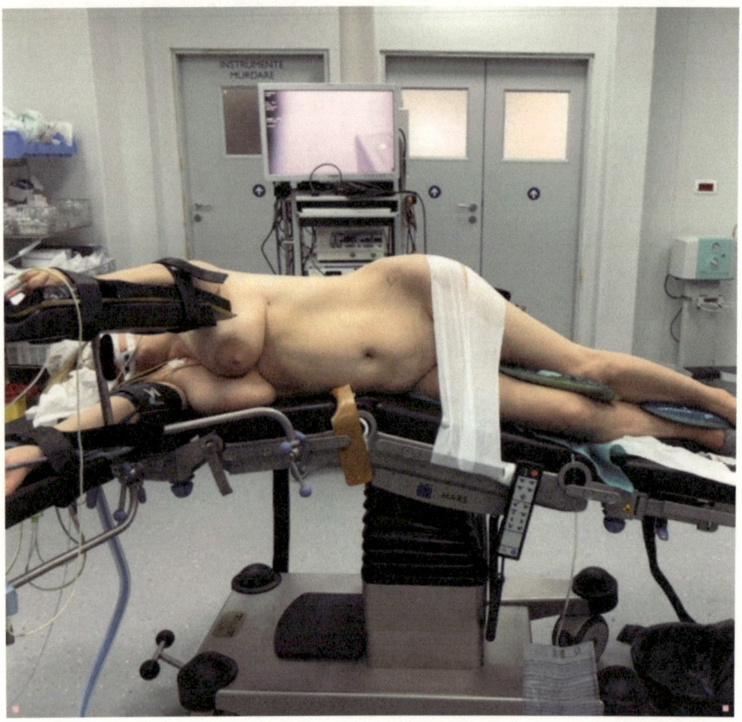

**Figure 20.**
*Position of the patient in sTEP L4 hernia repair.*

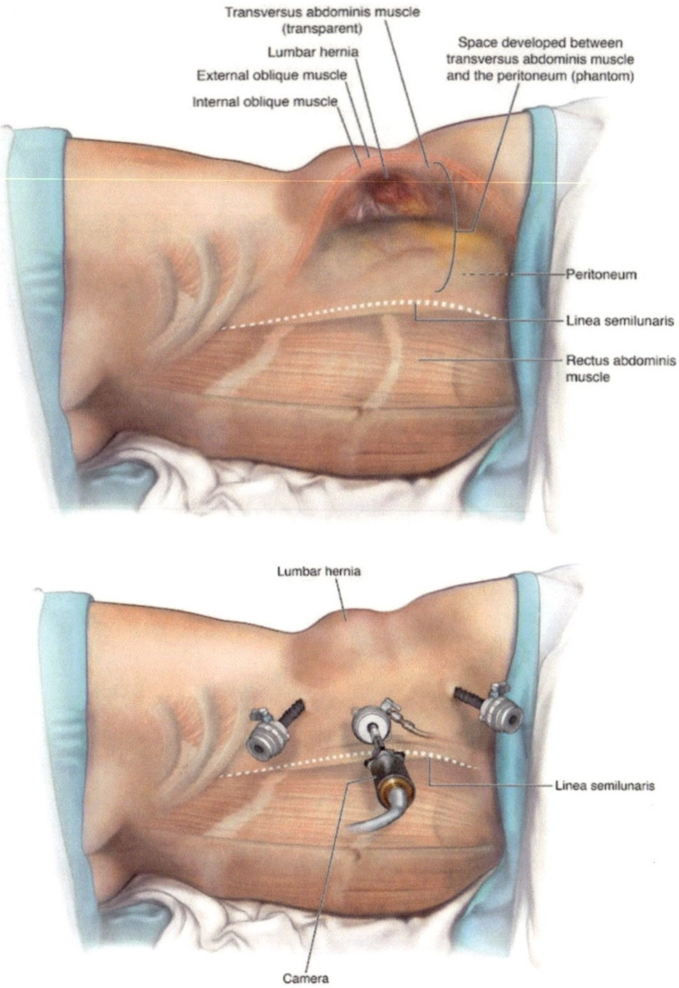


**Figure 21.**
*Development of the pretransversalis space, laterally to the linea semilunaris and port placement. (Courtesy of Dr. Jorge Daes).*

6. Slow exsufflation, under direct vision, allows us to ensure the mesh remains in the correct position

A different approach is performed for lumbar hernia repair (L4).

The position of the patient is on lateral decubitus, and the table is also flexed to increase the distance between the costal margin and the iliac crest (**Figure 20**).

The landmark for port placement is also lateral edge of the rectus muscle, but the ports will be placed laterally to this line.

The aim is to develop the retromuscular space without penetration into peritoneal cavity, close the defect, and place a mesh outside of the abdominal cavity (**Figure 21a** and **b**).

For that the key stages of the procedure are:

1. Insufflation of the peritoneal cavity and placing a port inside, in the hypochondrium, to identify the rectus muscle.

2. Development of preperitoneal pretransversalis space and port placement.

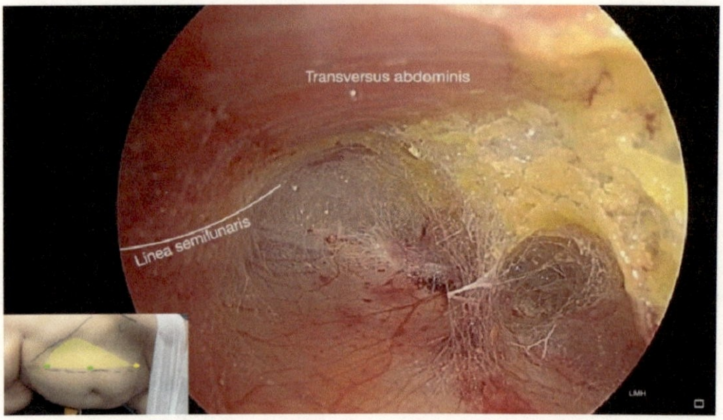


**Figure 22.**
*Pretransversalis space, laterally to the linea semilunaris.*

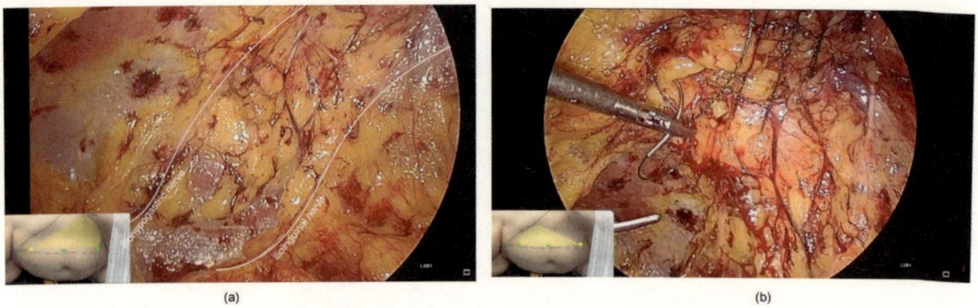


**Figure 23.**
*(a) Iliohypogastric and ilioinguinal nerves must be protected during dissection in the lumbar region. (b) closure of the defect.*

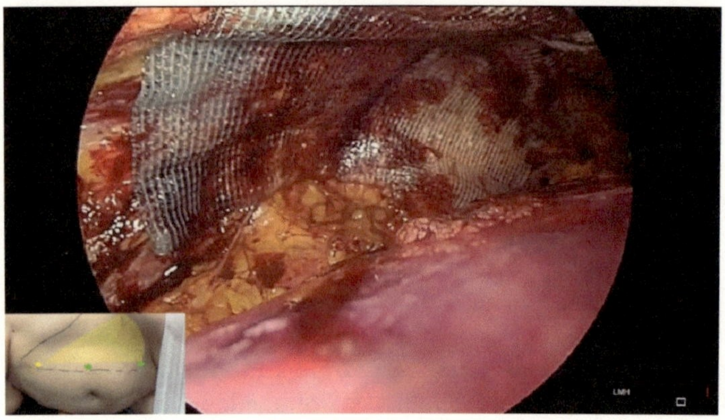

**Figure 24.**
*Mesh placement.*

Under direct vision, a second port is placed laterally to the semilunaris line and preperitoneally, and the gas to this port is connected to develop the preperitoneal space. An optic port is useful at this step.

The third port is placed also under direct vision, laterally to the semilunaris line.

Now, keeping the first port site will retract this port from the peritoneal cavity and change its direction laterally, in the preperitoneal space already created (**Figure 22**).

3. Dissection and closure of the defect (**Figure 23a** and **b**)

It is very important to understand the retroperitoneal lumbar anatomy, because during the retromuscular dissection, the iliohypogastric, ilioinguinal, and femoral-cutaneous nerves will come across and must be protected (**Figure 23**).

4. Mesh placement is the last step, respecting the overlap principle. Usually a self-gripping mesh is placed or a polypropylene mesh fixed with glue (**Figure 24**).

5. Slow exsufflation, under direct vision, allows us to ensure the mesh remains in the correct position.

### 3.3 Postoperative care

Soon postoperatively the patients are encouraged for an active mobilization. We do not recommend binders, but if the patients are more comfortable with binders, of course we accept to put it.

Coffee and chewing gum are recommended as soon as possible, and a liquid-semisolid diet is allowed for dinner. The level of pain after this surgery is usually very low. On our first study related to eTEP technique, we mentioned that in mean an eTEP patient gets 2.7 doses of painkiller (NSAI) for every 24 h of hospital stay.

The median length of hospitalization was in this study less than 24 hours postoperatively, even for eTEP-TAR cases. Usually the patients are discharged on the following day to their residence.

We began to actively asses the quality of life of our patients, and they filled out our questionnaire; in the study we published the results of questionnaires filled out by 42 from 60 patients which are expressed below:

In conclusion the eTEP techniques in ventral hernia repair (eRS and eTEP-TAR) combine the advantages of open retromuscular technique with the advantages of MIS.

## Author details

Victor G. Radu
Life Memorial Hospital, Medlife, Bucharest, Romania

*Address all correspondence to: dr.victor.radu@gmail.com

## References

[1] LeBlanc K, Allain Brent W. Jr. Laparoscopic Repair of Ventral Wall Abdominal Hernia - 3rd Edition: Prevention and Management [Online]. Available from: http://laparoscopy.blogs.com/prevention_management_3/2010/10/laparoscopic-repair-of-ventral-wall-abdominal-hernia.html. [Accessed: 02 September 2017]

[2] Bittner R et al. Guidelines for laparoscopic treatment of ventral and incisional abdominal wall hernias (International Endohernia Society (IEHS)-part 1). Surgical Endoscopy. Jan. 2014;**28**(1):2-29

[3] Miserez M, Penninckx F. Endoscopic totally preperitoneal ventral hernia repair. Surgical Endoscopy. Aug. 2002;**16**(8):1207-1213

[4] Schwarz J, Reinpold W, Bittner R. Endoscopic mini/less open sublay technique (EMILOS)—A new technique for ventral hernia repair. Langenbeck's Archives of Surgery. Feb. 2017;**402**(1):173-180

[5] Belyansky I, Zahiri HR, Park A. Laparoscopic transversus abdominis release, a novel minimally invasive approach to complex abdominal wall reconstruction. Surgical Innovation. Apr. 2016;**23**(2):134-141

[6] Belyansky I et al. A novel approach using the enhanced-view totally extraperitoneal (eTEP) technique for laparoscopic retromuscular hernia repair. Surgical Endoscopy. Sep, 2017;**32**:1531-1532

[7] Daes J. The enhanced view-totally extraperitoneal technique for repair of inguinal hernia. Surgical Endoscopy. Apr. 2012;**26**(4):1187-1189

[8] Novitsky YW. Posterior component separation via transversus abdominis muscle release: The TAR procedure. In: Hernia Surgery. Cham: Springer International Publishing; 2016. pp. 117-135

[9] Muysoms FE et al. Classification of primary and incisional abdominal wall hernias. Hernia. Aug. 2009;**13**(4):407-414

[10] Novitsky YW, editor. Hernia Surgery. Cham: Springer International Publishing; 2016

[11] De Keulenaer BL, De Waele JJ, Powell B, Malbrain MLNG. What is normal intra-abdominal pressure and how is it affected by positioning, body mass and positive end-expiratory pressure? Intensive Care Medicine. Jun. 2009;**35**(6):969-976

[12] Radu VG, Lica M. The Endoscopic Retromuscular Repair of Ventral Hernia: The eTEP Technique and Early Results. Hernia. 2019. DOI: 10.1007/s10029-019-01931-x/

Chapter 4

# Incisional Hernia

*Anil Kumar and Shiv Shankar Paswan*

## Abstract

Incisional hernia is one of the most common postoperative complications after abdominal surgery. Several studies have shown that incisional hernias have different etiologies which are related to the patient, the surgical technique, the suture material and experience of the surgeon. Most patients present with abdominal swelling with some level of discomfort, and in emergency the presentation is usually as bowel obstruction or strangulation which requires urgent exploration. The recurrence rate is almost the same for open as well as for laparoscopic approach. The hernia can be repaired either only by closing the defect with nonabsorbable suture or by applying mesh. The recurrence is very minimal with mesh application as compared to repair done only by suture. The mesh can be placed as onlay, inlay and in sublay positions. The intraperitoneal onlay mesh placement (IPOM) is the widely used laparoscopic method for the incisional hernia repair. The incisional hernia with larger defect usually more than 15 cm requires component separation to reconstruct the abdominal wall by releasing the external oblique or transverse abdominal muscle. The outcome of incisional hernia repair is dependent on the associated comorbid conditions like chronic cough, constipation, stricture of the urethra, benign prostate hyperplasia, ascites and obesity.

**Keywords:** incisional, hernia, mesh, laparotomy, component separation

## 1. Introduction

It is documented that in the first century A.D., a Roman doctor named Aulus Cornelius described the closure of the abdominal wall and elaborated a detailed description of the pre- and postoperative care of the patient [1]. Later on, another famous Roman-Greek physician, Galen, provided a detailed description of the mass closure of the abdominal wall and described the significance of paramedian incision in order to prevent incisional hernia [2]. The advancement of technology like the advent of modern anesthesia and antiseptic and upgradation of skills in the field of surgery in the present era promotes laparotomy. On the other hand, along with increased number of laparotomy, the incidence of incisional hernia also increased consequently. Incisional hernia is a frequent long-term complication of abdominal surgeries with a reported incidence of 2–20% [3–8]. In the USA alone, approximately 348,000 incisional hernia repairs are performed per year with total estimated procedural costs of $3.2 billion for ventral hernia repair [9–13]. Incisional hernia is more common than primary abdominal wall hernia, and both of these types are included in ventral hernia.

## 2. Surgical anatomy

The abdominal wall consists of the skin, fascia (Camper's and Scarpa's fascia), muscles (external oblique, internal oblique, transverse abdominis), rectus sheath,

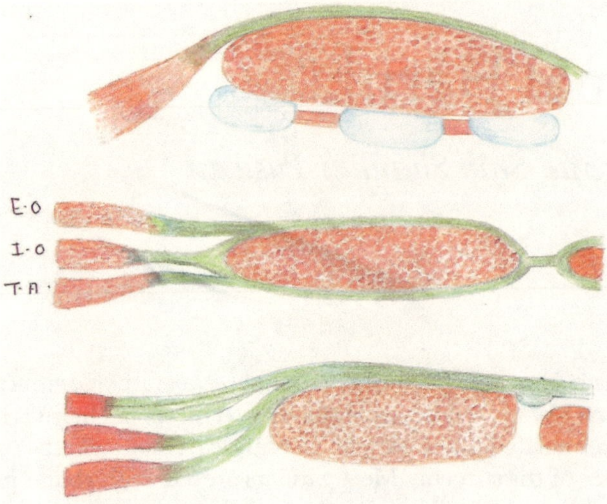


**Figure 1.**
*Rectus sheath formation.*

aponeurosis, linea alba, ligaments, openings, rings, blood vessels and nerves. **Figure 1** showed the formation of rectus sheath at three different levels on the abdominal wall. Above the costal margins, only the external oblique muscle with its aponeurosis forms the rectus sheath. In between xiphisternum and umbilicus, the external oblique remains in front, but the internal oblique splits to enclose the rectus muscles. The transverse abdominis is behind the internal oblique (**Figure 1**). All these muscles fuse to form the linea alba in the midline. The rectus abdominis muscles run vertically on either side of the linea alba. This area between the xiphisternum and umbilicus is the strongest area as compared to above the costal margin or below the semilunar line. Below the semilunar line, all the three aponeurosis are anterior to the rectus muscle and fuse in the midline to form the linea alba. So posterior rectus sheath is absent below the semilunar line, and that is why incisional hernias are more common below the umbilicus. On the other hand, the linea alba is the strongest layer of abdominal wall and less likely to develop incisional hernia if it has repaired properly with good bites through the linea alba.

The umbilicus is usually situated in the midline at the level of the superior iliac spine or at the level between the third and fourth lumbar vertebrae. The umbilicus is a strong fibrous ring. Hernia through the umbilicus may occur in children, obese patient and in multiparous women due to childhood umbilical infection, weak muscles and stretching of muscles due to repeated pregnancies, respectively.

## 3. Risk factors of incisional hernia

The development of incisional hernia is multifactorial. It may be related to the patient, surgical technique and experience of the surgeon, type of disease for which the incision was given or biological factors. **Table 1** summarized the various risk factors for the development of incisional hernia.

### 3.1 Patient-related factors

The incisional hernias are more common in the elderly age group because of multifactorial reasons including weak abdominal muscles, occurrence of comorbidity

| |
|---|
| **Patient-related factors:** |
| Age more than 60 years |
| Gender: female after cesarean section |
| Smoking |
| Socioeconomic condition: low profile |
| Occupation: lifting heavy weight |
| Comorbidities: diabetes mellitus, chronic cough, benign hypertrophy of the prostate, stricture of the urethra, chronic constipation, ascites, obstructive jaundice, chronic renal failure and certain connective tissue diseases (Marfan's syndrome, osteogenesis imperfecta and Ehlers-Danlos syndrome) |
| Post-organ transplant patient on immunosuppressive agents/corticosteroids |
| Obesity: (BMI >25 kg/m$^2$) |
| **Technical factors related to the surgical technique:** |
| Wrongly placed incision: lumbar incision, subcostal incision, lower midline incision and large transverse incision |
| Wound has not been approximated appropriately |
| Low surgical skill to close the abdomen |
| Strength and length of suture used is not appropriate |
| **Disease-related factors:** |
| Emergency operations |
| Type of surgery: bowel surgery, abdominal aortic aneurism, stoma closure, operations for peritonitis |
| Re-laparotomy |
| Wound infection |
| Long operating time |
| Increased blood loss |
| Damaged control surgery in trauma |
| Open abdomen: in the case of severe septicaemia, chance of abdominal compartment syndrome |
| **Biological factors:** |
| Nutritional deficiencies |
| Collagen and metalloproteinase synthesis |

**Table 1.**
*Risk factors of incisional hernia.*

like DM, malignancies and poor immunity. A BMI > 24.5 kg/m$^2$ is considered as an important risk factor for the development of incisional hernia [14–21]. The patient with low socioeconomic profile is more prone to develop incisional hernia because of malnourishment and being bound to lift heavy weight. Comorbidities like diabetes mellitus, malignancies, chronic lung diseases, benign hypertrophy of the prostate, chronic constipation as well as heavy weight lifting are well-known risk factors for hernia development by increasing the intra-abdominal pressure and delaying the wound healing. The use of immunosuppressant and steroids in organ transplant and other chronic disease patients increases the rate of wound infection, wound dehiscence and incisional hernia [22–27]. Smoking increases the risk of the development of incisional hernia by decreasing the blood flow and tissue oxygenation as well as collagen deposition in the surgical wound, and all these increase the infection rate and synergistically the incisional hernia as well [28, 29]. Abstinence from smoking 30 days preoperatively reduces the adverse effects of smoking on wound healing significantly. This emphasized the contributing role of smoking in causing incisional hernia [30, 31].

### 3.2 Technical factors related to the surgical technique

Despite advancements in techniques for abdominal wall closure, the incisional hernia rate following laparotomy is as high 15–20% [32]. Poor surgical technique may result in wound dehiscence and delay the wound healing. During closure of fascial edges, if it is not approximated properly, not using the suture with appropriate length and strength, then definitely in the postoperative period, there is a chance of wound dehiscence and development of incisional hernia especially if other predisposing factors are also present [33–35]. The preferably paramedian, oblique and transverse incisions are better than midline, large transverse, subcostal and lumbar incisions to prevent the occurrence of incisional hernia [36–39].

### 3.3 Disease-related factors

Wound infection and wound dehiscence are the major risk factors for the development of incisional hernia [18, 29, 35–37, 40–45]. Cases operated for infected intra-abdominal conditions like perforation peritonitis, gangrene of the intestine, severe necrotizing pancreatitis, etc. usually develop incisional hernia. The incidence of infection is less in a diabetic patient if their perioperative glycaemic control is adequate [46]. Furthermore, chance of infection in diabetic patient is higher than nondiabetic patient even after controlling for hyperglycaemia [47]. Re-laparotomy is a strong risk factor for IH [29]. Incidence of incisional hernias in open abdomen for severe septicaemia or for damaged control surgery ranged from 21% at 21 months to 54% after 5 years of follow-up [48–50]. Burst abdomen and open abdomen after the damage control surgery are the most important factors for the occurrence of incisional hernia. In the case of long operative time and where blood loss is more, the chance of IH development is also more. Incisional hernia has been also reported after traumatic abdominal injury [51]. Emergency surgeries are also associated with a higher incidence of incisional hernia development.

### 3.4 Biological factors

Apart from obesity, malnourishment is also the contributing factor for the development of incisional hernia by causing delayed wound healing and wound dehiscence [52–54]. Defective collagen metabolism with reduced ratio of collagen I-collagen III as well as a reduced ratio of matrix metalloproteinase 1 (MMP1)-MMP2 plays an important role in the development of IH [55]. Micronutrients like copper and zinc are required for the synthesis of the enzyme lysyl oxidase, and this enzyme is very important for the integrity of collagen molecule. So deficiency of these elements may cause the incisional hernia to occur. The plasminogen activator inhibitor, urokinase plasminogen activator inhibitor, in the scar tissue may contribute in the development of IH [56–58].

## 4. Classification

Various classifications for ventral hernia are available in literature, but unfortunately none of them have been widely accepted. Various classification systems are proposed by Chevrel and Rath, Korenkov et al., Schumpelick et al., Dietz et al., Ammaturo and Bassi and Miserez et al. [59–64]. They all have used variables like size and number of hernia defects, size of hernia sac and its ratio with anterior abdominal wall, primary or incisional hernia, recurrent hernia, location of hernia, and other symptoms and risk factors, in various combinations. To make it standardized, European Hernia Society (EHS) has divided the abdominal wall hernia as "Primary abdominal wall hernia" which is also called as ventral hernia and other "Incisional hernia" rather than either term. Recurrent hernia after treatment for primary abdominal wall hernia would fall in the group of incisional hernia. According to this system, classification of incisional hernias uses localisation and size of hernia as the two variables, as shown in **Table 2**. To avoid confusion with primary abdominal wall hernias (small, medium and large), a coded taxonomy was chosen ($W1 < 4$ cm; $W2 \geq 4$–10 cm; $W3 \geq 10$ cm) instead of a nominative one, and yes or no is used for the recurrent incisional hernia in EHS **Table 2**.

| EHS Incisional hernia classification | | | | |
|---|---|---|---|---|
| **Midline** | Subxiphoidal | | M1 | |
| | Epigastric | | M2 | |
| | Umbilical | | M3 | |
| | Infraumbilical | | M4 | |
| | Suprapubic | | M 5 | |
| **Lateral** | Subcostal | | L1 | |
| | Flank | | L2 | |
| | Iliac | | L3 | |
| | Lumbar | | L4 | |
| **Recurrent** | | **Incisional Hernia?** | **Yes** | **No** |
| | **Length** | Cm | **Width** | Cm |
| | **Width** | W1 < 4 cm | W2 ≥ 4–10 cm | W3 ≥ 10 cm |
| | **cm** | 0 | 0 | 0 |

**Table 2.**
*Showing EHS classification of incisional hernia.*

Here the abdomen was divided into a midline zone and a lateral zone.
The borders of the midline area are defined as follows:

1. Cranial: the xiphoid

2. Caudal: the pubic bone

3. Lateral: the lateral margin of the rectal sheath

Thus, all incisional hernias between the lateral margins of both rectus muscle sheaths are classified as midline hernias. A simple and easily memorable classification from M1 to M5 going from the xiphoid to the pubic bone is summarized in **Figure 2a**. Therefore, we define 5 M zones as follows:

1. M1: subxiphoidal (from the xiphoid till 3 cm caudally)

2. M2: epigastric (from 3 cm below the xiphoid till 3 cm above the umbilicus)

3. M3: umbilical (from 3 cm above till 3 cm below the umbilicus)

4. M4: infraumbilical (from 3 cm below the umbilicus till 3 cm above the pubis)

5. M5: suprapubic (from the pubic bone till 3 cm cranially).

Lateral hernias: The borders of the lateral area are defined as in **Figure 2b**:

1. Cranial: the costal margin

2. Caudal: the inguinal region

3. Medially: the lateral margin of the rectal sheath

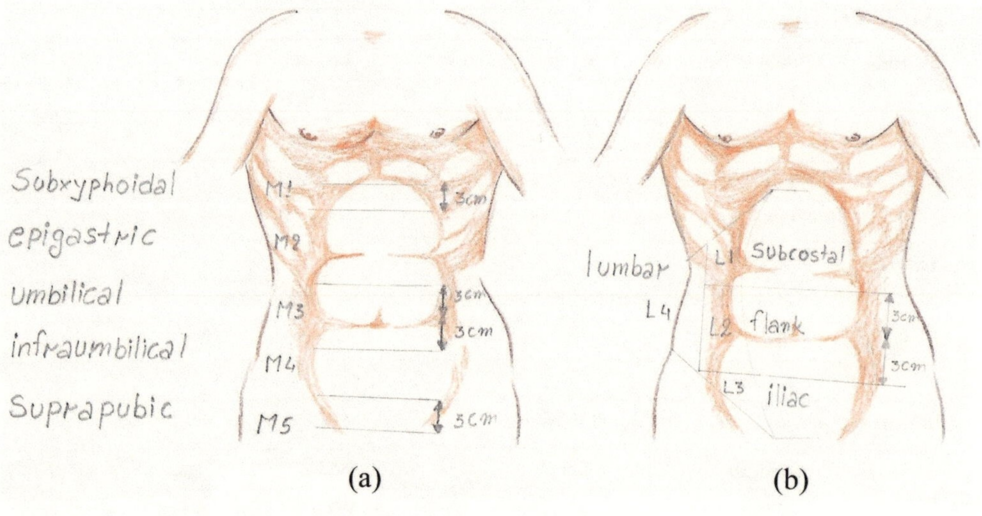


**Figure 2.**
*(a) 5M zone of incisional hernia. (b) 4L zone of incisional hernia.*

4. Laterally: the lumbar region

Thus, 4L zones on each side are defined as follows:

1. L1: subcostal (between the costal margin and a horizontal line 3 cm above the umbilicus)

2. L2: flank (lateral to the rectal sheath in the area 3 cm above and below the umbilicus)

3. L3: iliac (between a horizontal line 3 cm below the umbilicus and the inguinal region)

4. L4: lumbar (latero-dorsal of the anterior axillary line)

## 5. Clinical features

- History of surgery in the past.

- History of infection during the first surgery, postoperative cough, constipation, etc. is usually present.

- Serosanguinous discharge on the fourth postoperative day through the main suture line is a signal of the development of partial or total wound dehiscence. Such cases later develop an incisional hernia.

- Burst abdomen and open abdomen are more likely to develop incisional hernia (**Figure 3**).

- There is bulge or swelling around the scar (**Figure 4**).

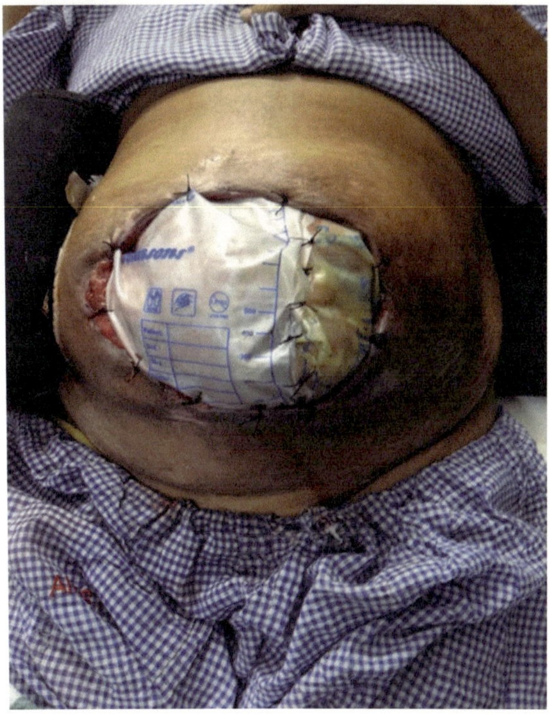

**Figure 3.**
*Burst abdomen prone to develop incisional hernia.*

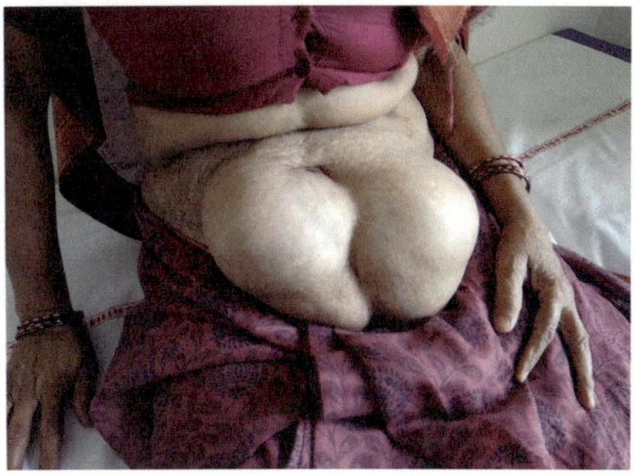

**Figure 4.**
*Complex Hernia with visible bulge.*

- The scar is thin and evidence of secondary changes like ulceration or skin color changes may be present (**Figure 5**).
- Expansile impulse on cough and reducibility may be present.
- Intraoperatively during creation of pneumoperitoneum, the bulge/swelling through the scar becomes more obvious (**Figure 6**).
- After reduction of the contents, a defect can be palpated through the scar. Defect depends upon the number of stiches that have given away.

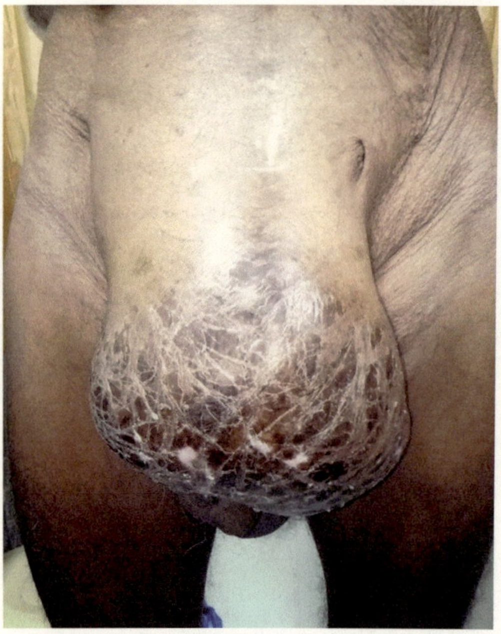

**Figure 5.**
*Lower abdominal wall hernia hanging up to the scrotum with secondary changes.*

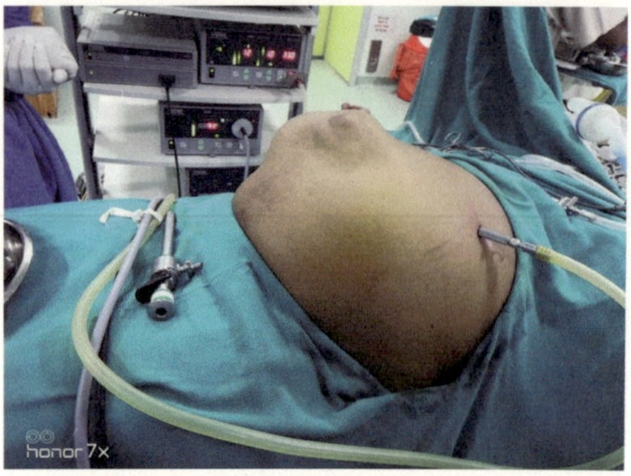


**Figure 6.**
*Prominent hernial defect after pneumoperitoneum.*

- In case of obstructed or impacted content in the defect, the patient may complain of pain in that area.
- Features of bowel obstruction or strangulation may be found in complicated cases.
- In most people, hernias limit patients' physical activities either due to the associated symptoms or as a precaution to avoid worsening.

### 5.1 Abdominal palpation

In most of the cases, hernial content can be palpated. In few cases even the edges of hernial defect can be appreciated, and the size can be measured. Except in obstructed and strangulated hernia, impulse on coughing and reducibility are present.

### 5.2 Percussion

Percussion guides us to assess whether the content of the hernia sac is solid, liquid or gas.

### 5.3 Auscultation

If the content of the sac is bowel loop, a peristaltic bowel sound may be heard and confirm the content of sac as bowel loop.

## 6. Evaluation

Although most cases of an incisional hernia are diagnosed with a history and physical examination, imaging is sometimes indicated in early stages, obese patients, or complex cases especially to outline the extent of defect and plan the surgical procedure. The first imaging modality in case of incisional hernia is ultrasonography, but the computed tomography scan (CT) is the most commonly used method for the diagnosis as well as for planning of operative management especially for complex cases [65, 66]. CT scan evaluates the incisional hernia by confirming its diagnosis, sizing the defect, identifying the hernia content and assessing the abdominal cavity to plan the surgical treatment. Magnetic resonance imaging (MRI) can also be used to assess abdominal wall hernias but are less commonly used for academic purpose only.

## 7. Management

The management of incisional hernia includes nonoperative and operative management. Nonoperative management is indicated in patients who are not fit for surgery, those who require preoperative optimization or those who have highly complex hernia like loss of abdominal wall domain, patient with diagnosis of metastatic cancer, advanced cirrhosis, severe cardiopulmonary disease and super obesity (BMI $\geq$ 50 kg/m$^2$).

### 7.1 Preoperative management

1. Weight reduction is very important before operating for incisional hernia. It is required to bring the BMI < 30–40 Kg/m$^2$.

2. Control of COPD, definitive treatment of benign prostatic hyperplasia, stricture of the urethra and all other conditions who may increase the intra-abdominal pressure in postoperative period in view to avoid the recurrence.

3. Cessation of smoking is very helpful for good outcome.

### 7.2 Indication of surgery in incisional hernia

1. To get the relief from symptoms

2. Prevention of complication like pain, incarceration, bowel obstruction and strangulation

3. To improve the quality of life

There are various operations for the treatment of incisional hernia depending upon the size of the defect, location of the hernia, patient choice as per their economical conditions as laparoscopic repair may be costly and surgeon expertise. **Table 3** summarized the different surgical options for incisional hernia.

### 7.3 Open hernia repair

Although minimal invasive surgery is widely acceptable and treatment of choice in present era, but open surgery still plays a very important role in incisional hernia repair especially in conditions contraindicated for laparoscopic surgery like very large, non-reducible hernia and strangulated hernia. Besides these contraindicated cases, for small umbilical hernias, open repair is preferred choice. Open repair can be done either by suture repair or by applying mesh. Recurrence rate after suture repair is 42% and after mesh repair only 24%. Ideally if the defect size is more than 4 cm, mesh placement should be the preferred approach, but even for the smaller defect which is less than 2 cm in size, the recurrence rate is 5.6% with suture method as compared to mesh where only 2.2% recurrence rate occurs. Three main positions of the mesh placement for incisional hernia are onlay, inlay and sublay positions (**Figure 3**).

Onlay mesh is placed over the anterior fascia and under the subcutaneous tissue. Inlay mesh is placed to the margin of the aponeurosis. In this case the mesh acts as bridge between the two fascial edges. Sublay mesh is placed retro muscularly and preperitoneally. The sublay mesh placement has been reported to be the best regarding recurrence and skin and soft tissue infection but is associated with higher risk of chronic pain. The main principle to place the mesh is that the mesh should be overlapped at least 5 cm all around the defect. Otherwise, the plane is created between the posterior rectus sheath and rectus muscle, and the mesh is placed in that location, and the anterior rectus sheath is sutured. This is called retro muscular sublay mesh repair. Before placing the mesh, the sac is opened, the greater omentum is excised, and the content is reduced followed by closure of the peritoneum. A mesh is kept in place. In all these repairs, tensionless, nonabsorbable suture repairs are done. Seroma formation is a common complication in open mesh repair which can be overcome by placing drain before closing the wound.

| |
|---|
| **Open hernia repair** |
| Suture repair |
| Mesh repair |
| **Laparoscopic incisional hernia repair** |
| Primary fascial closure |
| Different mesh fixation techniques |
| **Abdominal wall reconstruction technique** |
| Bridge repair |
| Anterior component separation (ACS) |
| Perforator-sparing ACS |
| Endoscopic ACS |
| Posterior component separation |
| **Preoperative tissue expansion** |
| Tissue expanders |
| Progressive pneumoperitoneum |
| **Flap and tissue transfer** |

**Table 3.**
*Surgical options for incisional hernia repair.*

### 7.4 Laparoscopic incisional hernia repair

First time in 1993, LeBlanc and Booth introduced the laparoscopic method for incisional hernia repair [67], and since then various studies and approach have been published in literature [68]. Laparoscopic repair of incisional hernia is a very safe procedure and having all the advantages of minimal access surgery like earlier recovery, decreased hospital stay and less wound infections. It has been reported to have a low conversion rate of 2.4%, an enterotomy rate of 1.8% and recurrence rate of 4.2%; however recent randomized trials have shown a similar recurrence in laparoscopic and open hernia repair.

### 7.5 Contraindications of laparoscopic incisional hernia repair

Contraindications to laparoscopic incisional hernia repair are almost the same as for other laparoscopic surgeries which are summarized in **Table 4**.

### 7.6 Operative steps of laparoscopic incisional hernia repair

1. Complete all the preanaesthetic checkup and preoperative order like Nil per orally 12 hours prior to surgery and securing IV line for fluid administration, antibiotic test dose and shifting the patient to the operation room.

2. Take the patient on the table in supine position, and after general anesthesia, pneumoperitoneum is created.

3. Three working ports are placed as far as possible from the scar of the previous abdominal surgeries.

4. Start the adhesiolysis if indicated and repose the sac content into the peritoneal cavity.

5. Primary fascial closure may be done to restore the normal anatomy. The technique for this primary fascial closure may be intracorporeal closure, extracorporeal closure or with the help of suture passing needle. This step prevents the postoperative bulge and seroma formation. It also allows wider lateral mesh overlap, thereby preventing recurrence.

6. Overlap of mesh should be ideally 5 cm in all directions because of significant postoperative shrinkage of mesh.

7. Before fixing the mesh, the intra-abdominal pressure should reduce to 5–8 mmHg, so that the abdominal wall is minimally stretched revealing the true size of the hernia defect.

8. Fixation of mesh is usually done by tacker or suture.

| |
|---|
| The larger defect is usually more than of 10–15 cm |
| Prior multiple open surgeries |
| Ascites with child class C cirrhosis |
| Inability to create a working space |

**Table 4.**
*Contraindications of laparoscopic incisional hernia repair.*

## 8. Abdominal wall reconstruction

The open and the laparoscopic techniques are used for small- and medium-sized defects but are not sufficient for very large defects which are too large to allow the fascial to be approximated. In such large size defect, a novel method of abdominal component separation was being developed. According to the EHS, large ventral hernia is defined as a hernia with defect greater than 10 cm and loss of domain defined by more than 50% of visceral contents lying chronically beyond the bounds of the abdomen. In such defect repair by open or laparoscopic method is usually not possible and component separation is required which was first introduced by Ramirez and colleagues in 1990 [69]. Component separation may be anterior, posterior, perforator-sparing ACS or endoscopic ACS.

### 8.1 Component separation

The component separation technique was first described by Ramirez in 1990. It is very effective for reconstructing large or complex midline abdominal wall defects, and it has the advantage of restoring the innervated dynamic abdominal wall integrity without producing undue tension on the repair. It is a myofascial release that separates the components of the abdominal wall allowing their mobilization into adjacent tissue defects. Classic CST involves releasing the rectus muscle from its posterior sheath and releasing the aponeurosis of the external oblique muscle along the lateral side of the rectus, allowing the rectus muscle to slide towards the midline with its attached internal oblique and anterior rectus fascia. In fact this is called anterior component separation. Fascial defects up to 10 cm wide at the upper abdomen, 20 cm at the waistline and 6 cm at the suprapubic region may be closed using this method.

#### *8.1.1 Steps of anterior component separation*

1. Through a laparotomy incision, the posterior rectus sheath is cleared bilaterally of any attachments to the viscera through careful lysis of adhesions.

2. The rectus muscle is loosely attached to its posterior sheath and can be freed from the posterior sheath at this point, as Ramirez did. Freeing the rectus muscle from its posterior sheath allows advancement of this muscle by 3 cm in the upper third, 5 cm in the middle third and 3 cm in the lower third.

3. Separate the skin and subcutaneous tissues from the anterior rectus sheath using electrocautery. Develop this plane until about 2 cm beyond the lateral edge of the rectus sheath. Further lateral dissection in patients with limited subcutaneous tissue may place the resulting skin flaps at risk for ischemia and failure resulting in a large soft tissue defect that will require split-thickness skin grafting.

4. Carefully incise the external oblique aponeurosis 2 cm lateral to the lateral edge of the rectus sheath. Extend this incision parallel to the rectus muscle, superiorly advancing at least 5–7 cm above the costal margin and inferiorly down to the suprapubic region. The plane between the external and internal oblique aponeuroses is relatively avascular and should be bluntly dissected free down to the mid to posterior axillary line.

#### *8.1.2 Complications of ACS*

The surgical site infection (SSI), site dehiscence, seroma, hematoma, site necrosis and recurrences have been reported to be highest with ACS compared to other component separation techniques.

### 8.2 Posterior component separation

In order to gain further mobility of the rectus sheath, Crbonell et al. introduced the concept of posterior component separation (PCS) which involved extending the retro muscular plane laterally between the internal oblique and transverse abdominis. Further modification of the technique was done by Novinsky et al. with the release of transverse abdominis muscle and entry into the retro rectus space, and dissection is carried till lateral of psoas muscle, avoiding skin flap necrosis. A mesh is placed in sublay position after closing the posterior rectus sheath in the midline. PCS is the CS procedure of choice to obtain medial fascial advancement and the creation of huge space for the mesh placement.

#### *8.2.1 Steps of PCS*

An incision is made in the posterior rectus sheath within 0.5 cm of its medial border. This incision is extended superiorly and inferiorly along the entire length of the rectus muscle. Dissection is continued medial to lateral as blunt or sharp preventing injury to the epigastric vessels as it lies within the muscles. The lateral limit of this dissection in PCS is the linea semilunaris up to the lateral border of the rectus muscle, the area of fusion of the anterior and posterior rectus sheaths. It is important to identify and preserve intercostal neurovascular structures entering the posterior aspect of the rectus muscle. Superiorly, this plane extends to the retroxiphoid/retrosternal space and inferiorly into the space of Retzius. In many circumstances, dissection in the retrorectus space up to the linea semilunaris is insufficient to permit adequate abdominal wall reconstruction, and there is also insufficient retrorectus space to permit adequate prosthetic reinforcement for hernia. In order to extend the retrorectus dissection lateral to the linea semilunaris, intramuscular dissection is possible by diving the internal oblique muscle; further dissection is performed within the preperitoneal plane or with transverse abdominis release (TAR). Incision is made approximately 0.5 cm medial to the linea semilunaris in the posterior sheath to expose the transverse muscle. It is easy in the upper half of the abdomen where the muscle belly is well developed. With electrocautery, transection of the transverse abdominis muscle is done to prevent injury to the transversalis fascia or peritoneum. This plane may extend superiorly beyond the costal margin to the diaphragm, inferiorly to the myopectineal orifice and laterally to the psoas muscle. Similarly, TAR is completed on the contralateral side. This is followed by reconstruction of the posterior layer with re-approximation of the posterior rectus sheath in midline using running suture. A large mesh is used to cover the space created at the retro muscular space up to the lateral border of dissection. The anterior rectus sheath is approximated in the midline.

## 9. Preoperative tissue expansion

In situations where fascial closure cannot be achieved even after CS, several other options have been described, each with its own advantages and disadvantages.

Hybrid Operation have been described where fascia is partially closed & reminder is bridge with an absorbable mesh in underlay or sublay position. Addition of vacuum-assisted closure to reduce the SSO and SSI in hybrid procedures has also been described. An alternative to these procedures is preoperative tissue expansion or flap and tissue transfer.

## 10. Tissue expanders

Tissue expanders are used to provide soft tissue coverage and restore abdominal domain by increasing both the size and the vascularity of the donor tissue by producing a strong, vascularized capsule around the expanders. Various sites of placing tissue expanders have been described like in the subcutaneous space, abdominal wall intramuscular spaces (between the internal oblique and transverse abdominis muscles), intermuscular sites (between the external and internal oblique muscles) and finally intra-abdominally. The expanders can be insufflated over various weeks depending on patient tolerance. Before starting filling of the expander, a period of wound healing is usually awaited for 3 weeks to prevent expander exclusion. Expanded skin retracts after removal of expanders, hence overexpansion is necessary. Complications like expulsion, exposure or infection of implants can occur in about 15% cases.

## 11. Progressive pneumoperitoneum

Reduction of contents of giant hernias may result in abdominal compartment syndrome. Progressive pneumoperitoneum technique is used to stretch the abdominal wall muscles before repair. Progressive pneumoperitoneum (PPP) increases the capacity of the retracted abdominal cavity, performs a pneumatic lysis of intestinal adhesions, allows the reduction of the hernia contents and improves diaphragmatic function. Air, $CO_2$ or NO is insufflated over a period of a few weeks every couple of days to about a total of 15–20 L depending on patient tolerability monitored by the development of scapular pain, dyspnoea or subcutaneous emphysema. Once tissue expansion is obtained, hernia repair is attempted.

## 12. Flap and tissue transfer

An alternative to tissue expansion is the use of plastic surgery procedures of flap and tissue transfer like latissimus dorsi, tensor fascia lata or rectus femoris flaps, but they are more complex and result in donor site defects and functional limitations.

## Author details

Anil Kumar[1]* and Shiv Shankar Paswan[2]

1 All India Institute of Medical Sciences, Patna, India

2 All India Institute of Medical Sciences, Bhubaneswar, India

*Address all correspondence to: dranil4@gmail.com

## References


[1] Papavramidou NS, Christopoulou-Aletras H. Treatment of "hernia" in the writings of Celsus (first century AD). World Journal of Surgery. 2005;**10**:1343-1347

[2] Sanders DL, Kingsnorth AN. From ancient to contemporary times: A concise history of incisional hernia repair. Hernia. 2012;**16**:1-7

[3] Hodgson NC, Malthaner RA, Ostbye T. The search for an ideal method of abdominal fascial closure: A metaanalysis. Annals of Surgery. 2000;**231**(3):436-442

[4] Eisner L, Harder F. Incisional hernias. Der Chirurg. 1997;**68**(4):304-309

[5] Klinge U, Prescher A, Klosterhalfen B, Schumpelick V. Development and pathophysiology of abdominal wall defects. Der Chirurg. 1997;**68**(4):293-303

[6] Mudge M, Hughes LE. Incisional hernia: A 10-year prospective study of incidence and attitudes. The British Journal of Surgery. 1985;**72**(1):70-71

[7] Santora TA, Roslyn JJ. Incisional hernia. The Surgical Clinics of North America. 1993;**73**(3):557-570

[8] Schumpelick V, Klinge U, Welty G. Meshes within the abdominal wall. Der Chirurg. 1999;**70**(8):876-887

[9] National Center for Health Statistics. Combined Surgery Data (NHDS and NSAS) Data Highlights. 1996. Available from: http://www.cdc.gov/nchs/about/major/hdasd/combtab.htm

[10] Franz MG, Kuhn MA, Nguyen K, Wang X, Ko F, Wright TE, et al. Transforming growth factor beta (2) lowers the incidence of incisional hernias. The Journal of Surgical Research. 2001;**97**(2):109-116

[11] Rutkow IM. Demographic and socioeconomic aspects of hernia repair in the United States in 2003. The Surgical Clinics of North America. 2003;**5**:1045-1051

[12] Flum DR, Horvath K, Koepsell T. Have outcomes of incisional hernia repair improved with time? A population-based analysis. Annals of Surgery. 2003;**237**:129-135

[13] Poulose BK, Shelton J, Phillips S, Moore D, Nealon W, Penson D, et al. Epidemiology and cost of ventral hernia repair: Making the case for hernia research. Hernia. 2012;**16**:179-183

[14] Llaguna OH, Avgerinos DV, Lugo JZ, Matatov T, Abbadessa B, Martz JE, et al. Incidence and risk factors for the development of incisional hernia following elective laparoscopic versus open colon resections. American Journal of Surgery. 2010;**200**:265-269

[15] Manninen MJ, Lavonius M, Perhoniemi VJ. Results of incisional hernia repair. A retrospective study of 172 unselected hernioplasties. The European Journal of Surgery. 1991;**157**:29-31

[16] Sugerman HJ, Kellum JM Jr, Reines HD, DeMaria EJ, Newsome HH, Lowry JW. Greater risk of incisional hernia with morbidly obese than steroid-dependent patients and low recurrence with prefascial polypropylene mesh. American Journal of Surgery. 1996;**171**:80-84

[17] Veljkovic R, Protic M, Gluhovic A, Potic Z, Milosevic Z, Stojadinovic A. Prospective clinical trial of factors predicting the early development of incisional hernia after midline laparotomy. Journal of the American College of Surgeons. 2010;**210**:210-219

[18] Murray BW, Cipher DJ, Pham T, Anthony T. The impact of surgical site infection on the development of incisional hernia and small bowel obstruction in colorectal surgery. American Journal of Surgery. 2011;**202**:558-560

[19] Schreinemacher MH, Vijgen GH, Dagnelie PC, Bloemen JG, Huizinga BF, Bouvy ND. Incisional hernias in temporary stoma wounds: A cohort study. Archives of Surgery. 2011;**146**:94-99

[20] Lau B, Kim H, Haigh PI, Tejirian T. Obesity increases the odds of acquiring and incarcerating noninguinal abdominal wall hernias. The American Surgeon. 2012;**78**:1118-1121

[21] Sauerland S, Korenkov M, Kleinen T, Arndt M, Paul A. Obesity is a risk factor for recurrence after incisional hernia repair. Hernia. 2004;**8**:42-46

[22] Jargon D, Friebe V, Hopt UT, Obermaier R. Risk factors and prevention of incisional hernia–What is evidence-based? Zentralblatt für Chirurgie. 2008;**133**:453-457

[23] Koivukangas V, Oikarinen A, Risteli J, Haukipuro K. Effect of jaundice and its resolution on wound re-epithelization, skin collagen synthesis, and serum collagen propeptide levels in patients with neoplastic pancreaticobiliary obstruction. The Journal of Surgical Research. 2005;**124**:237-243

[24] Hesselink VJ, Luijendijk RW, de Wilt JH, Heide R, Jeekel J. An evaluation of risk factors in incisional hernia recurrence. Surgery, Gynecology & Obstetrics. 1993;**176**:228-234

[25] Aboian E, Winter DC, Metcalf DR, Wolff BG. Perineal hernia after proctectomy: Prevalence, risks, and management. Diseases of the Colon and Rectum. 2006;**49**:1564-1568

[26] Brewer MB, Rada EM, Milburn ML, Goldberg NH, Singh DP, Cooper M, et al. Human acellular dermal matrix for ventral hernia repair reduces morbidity in transplant patients. Hernia. 2011;**15**:141-145

[27] Janssen H, Lange R, Erhard J, Malagó M, Eigler FW, Broelsch CE. Causative factors, surgical treatment and outcome of incisional hernia after liver transplantation. The British Journal of Surgery. 2002;**89**:1049-1054

[28] Yang GP, Longaker MT. Abstinence from smoking reduces incisional wound infection: A randomized controlled trial. Annals of Surgery. 2003;**238**:6-8

[29] Sørensen LT, Hemmingsen UB, Kirkeby LT, Kallehave F, Jørgensen LN. Smoking is a risk factor for incisional hernia. Archives of Surgery. 2005;**140**:119-123

[30] Sørensen LT, Karlsmark T, Gottrup F. Abstinence from smoking reduces incisional wound infection: A randomized controlled trail. Annals of Surgery. 2003;**238**:1-5

[31] Frangou C. U.S. Panel of Surgeons Says 'No' to Noncompliant Hernia Patients. 2014. Available from: http://www.generalsurgerynews.com [Accessed: 12 August 2014]

[32] Söderbäck H, Gunnarsson U, Hellman P, Sandblom G. Incisional hernia after surgery for colorectal cancer: A population-based register study. International Journal of Colorectal Disease. 2018 Oct;**33**(10):1411-1417

[33] Berrevoet F. Prevention of incisional hernias after open abdomen treatment. Frontiers in Surgery. 2018;**5**:11

[34] Zucker BE, Simillis C, Tekkis P, Kontovounisios C. Suture choice to reduce occurrence of surgical site infection, hernia, wound dehiscence

and sinus/fistula: A network meta-analysis. Annals of the Royal College of Surgeons of England. 2019 Mar;**101**(3):150-161

[35] Müller-Riemenschneider F, Roll S, Friedrich M, Zieren J, Reinhold T, von der Schulenburg JM, et al. Medical effectiveness and safety of conventional compared to laparoscopic incisional hernia repair: A systematic review. Surgical Endoscopy. 2007;**21**:2127-2136

[36] Beltrán MA, Cruces KS. Incisional hernia after McBurney incision: Retrospective case-control study of risk factors and surgical treatment. World Journal of Surgery. 2008;**32**:596-601

[37] Le Huu NR, Mege D, Ouaïssi M, Sielezneff I, Sastre B. Incidence and prevention of ventral incisional hernia. Journal of Visceral Surgery. 2012;**149** (5 Suppl):e3-e14

[38] Bucknall TE, Cox PJ, Ellis H. Burst abdomen and incisional hernia: A prospective study of 1129 major laparotomies. British Medical Journal (Clinical Research Edition). 1982;**284**:931-933

[39] Bickenbach KA, Karanicolas PJ, Ammori JB, Jayaraman S, Winter JM, Fields RC, et al. Up and down or side to side? A systemic review and meta-analysis examining the impact of incision on outcomes after abdominal surgery. American Journal of Surgery. 2013;**206**:400-409

[40] Sanchez VM, Abi-Haidar YE, Itani KM. Mesh infection in ventral incisional hernia repair: Incidence, contributing factors, and treatment. Sugical Infections (Larchmt). 2011;**12**:205-210

[41] Brandl A, Laimer E, Perathoner A, Zitt M, Pratschke J, Kafka-Ritsch R. Incisional hernia rate after open abdomen treatment with negative pressure and delayed primary fascia closure. Hernia. 2014;**18**:105-111

[42] Song IH, Ha HK, Choi SG, Jeon BG, Kim MJ, Park KJ. Analysis of risk factors for the development of incisional and parastomal hernias in patients after colorectal surgery. Journal of the Korean Society of Coloproctology. 2012;**28**:299-303

[43] Gislason H, Viste A. Closure of burst abdomen after major gastrointestinal operations–Comparison of different surgical techniques and later development of incisional hernia. The European Journal of Surgery. 1999;**165**:958-961

[44] Lamont PM, Ellis H. Incisional hernia in re-opened abdominal incisions: An overlooked risk factor. The British Journal of Surgery. 1988;**75**:374-376

[45] Houck JP, Rypins EB, Sarfeh IJ, Juler GL, Shimoda KJ. Repair of incisional hernia. Surgery, Gynecology & Obstetrics. 1989;**169**: 397-399

[46] Dronge AS, Perkal MF, Kancir S, Concato J, Aslan M, Rosenthal RA. Long-term glycemic control and postoperative infectious complications. Archives of Surgery. 2006;**141**:375-380

[47] Martin ET, Kaye KS, Knott C, Nguyen H, Santarossa M, Evans R, et al. Diabetes and risk of surgical site infection: A systemic review and meta-analysis. Infection Control and Hospital Epidemiology. 2015;**37**:88-99

[48] Bjørsum-Meyer T, Skarbye M, Jensen KH. Vacuum with mesh is a feasible temporary closure device after fascial dehiscence. Danish Medical Journal. 2013;**60**(11):A4719. PubMed, Google Scholar

[49] Petersson U, Acosta S, Björck M. Vacuum-assisted wound

closure and mesh-mediated fascial traction—A novel technique for late closure of the open abdomen. World Journal of Surgery. 2007;**31**(11):2133-2137. DOI: 10.1007/s00268-007-9222-0. PubMed, CrossRef, Google Scholar

[50] Willms A, Güsgen C, Schaaf S, Bieler D, von Websky M, Schwab R. Management of the open abdomen using vacuum-assisted wound closure and mesh-mediated fascial traction. Langenbeck's Archives of Surgery. 2015;**400**(1):91-99. DOI: 10.1007/s00423-014-1240-4

[51] Yagnik VD, Joshipura V. Non-incisional traumatic lateral abdominal wall hernia. ANZ Journal of Surgery. 2017;**87**(11):952-953. IH after traumatic abdominal injury

[52] Daley J, Khuri SF, Henderson W, Hur K, Gibbs JO, Barbour G, et al. Risk adjustment of the postoperative morbidity rate for the comparative assessment of the quality of surgical care: Results of the National Veterans Affairs Surgical Risk Study. Journal of the American College of Surgeons. 1997;**185**:328-340

[53] Spencer RJ, Hayes KD, Rose S, Zhao Q, Rathouz PJ, Rice LW, et al. Risk factors for early-occurring and late-occurring incisional hernias after primary laparotomy for ovarian cancer. Obstetrics & Gynecology. 2015;**125**:407-413

[54] Jie B, Jiang ZM, Nolan MT, Zhu SN, Yu K, Kondrup J. Impact of preoperative nutritional support on clinical outcome in abdominal surgical patients at nutritional risk. Nutrition. 2012;**28**:1022-1027

[55] Bellón JM, Durán HJ. Biological factors involved in the genesis of incisional hernia. Cirugía Española. 2008;**83**:3-7

[56] Ozdemir S, Ozis ES, Gulpinar K, Aydin SM, Eren AA, Demirtas S, et al. The value of copper and zinc levels in hernia formation. European Journal of Clinical Investigation. 2011;**41**:285-290

[57] Salameh JR, Talbott LM, May W, Gosheh B, Vig PJ, McDaniel DO. Role of biomarkers in incisional hernias. The American Surgeon. 2007;**73**:561-567

[58] Rosch R, Binnebösel M, Junge K, Lynen-Jansen P, Mertens PR, Klinge U, et al. Analysis of c-myc, PAI-1 and uPAR in patients with incisional hernias. Hernia. 2008;**12**:285-288

[59] Chevrel JP, Rath AM. Classification of incisional hernias of the abdominal wall. Hernia. 2000;**4**:7-11

[60] Korenkov M, Paul A, Sauerland S, Neugebauer E, Arndt M, Chevrel JP, et al. Classification and surgical treatment of incisional hernia. Results of an experts' meeting. Langenbeck's Archives of Surgery. 2001;**386**:65-73

[61] Schumpelick V. Narbenhernie. In: Schumpelick V, editor. Hernien. Stuttgart: Thieme; 2000. pp. 266-269

[62] Dietz UA, Hamelmann W, Winkler MS, Debus ES, Malafaia O, Czeczko NG, et al. Journal of Plastic, Reconstructive & Aesthetic Surgery. 2007;**60**(4):383-388. PubMed

[63] Ammaturo C, Bassi G. The ratio between anterior abdominal wall surface/wall defect surface: A new parameter to classify abdominal incisional hernias. Hernia. 2005;**9**:316-321. PubMed

[64] Miserez M et al. The European hernia society groin hernia classification: Simple and easy to remember. Hernia. 2007;**11**(2):113-116

[65] Farukhi MA, Mattingly MS, Clapp B, Tyroch AH. CT scan reliability in detecting internal hernia after gastric bypass. Journal of the Society of

Laparoendoscopic Surgeons. 2017;**21**(4). PMC free article. PubMed

[66] Holihan JL, Karanjawala B, Ko A, Askenasy EP, Matta EJ, Gharbaoui L, et al. Use of computed tomography in diagnosing ventral hernia recurrence: A blinded, prospective, multispecialty evaluation. JAMA Surgery. 2016;**151**(1):7-13. PubMed

[67] LeBlanc KA, Booth WV, Whitaker JM, Bellanger DE. Laparoscopic incisional and ventral herniorrhaphy: Our initial 100 patients. Hernia. 2001;**5**:41-45. PubMed. Google Scholar

[68] Franklin ME, Gonzalez JJ, Glass JL, Manjarrez A. Laparoscopic ventral and incisional hernia repair: An 11-year experience. Hernia. 2004;**8**:23-27

[69] Ramirez OM, Ruas E, Dellon AL. "Components separation" method for closure of abdominal-wall defects: An anatomic and clinical study. Plastic and Reconstructive Surgery. 1990;**86**(3):519-526

Chapter 5

# Refinements and Advancements in Anterior Component Separation

*Sahil K. Kapur and Charles E. Butler*

## Abstract

This chapter will explore the newest innovations for performing anterior component separation (CS). It will include open CS, perforator sparing CS and minimally invasive component separation (MICS). It will also address the use of various meshes and their plane of inset. It will cover soft tissue management including panniculectomy, quilting sutures and drains. Fascial closure techniques will also be included. The highlight of this chapter will be the description of tips and tricks of performing MICS. We will also touch upon preoperative preparation such as body mass index (BMI) optimization and smoking cessation as well as management of postoperative complications including surgical site infections, skin necrosis and seroma.

**Keywords:** hernia, mesh, component separation, abdominal wall

## 1. Introduction

Abdominal wall domain and function is maintained by balancing the centripetal forces exerted on the abdominal wall by the internal organs with the centrifugal forces exerted by the combined action of the musculofascial abdominal wall. This musculoaponeurotic girdle consisting of a layered muscle arrangement coalescing into a static ligamentous supports can be broadly subdivided into the ventral abdominal wall and the lateral abdominal wall. The ventral abdominal wall comprises of longitudinally oriented rectus abdominis muscles encased in the anterior and posterior rectus sheath bounded centrally by the linea alba. It extends from the xiphoid process to the pubic symphysis. The lateral abdominal wall consists of a layered arrangement the external oblique, internal oblique, transversus abdominis and transversalis fascia. It extends from the costal margins superiorly to the iliac crest inferiorly and the linea semilunaris anteriorly to the thoracolumbar fascia posteriorly. The linea alba, linea semilunaris, and thoracolumbar fascia serve as a static attachment points for these muscles and translate their circumferentially and longitudinally oriented force vectors to generate centrifugal forces necessary to contain the internal organs and maintain abdominal wall domain.

The incidence of ventral or incisional hernia following laparotomy ranges from 1 to 20% [1–3], while the recurrence rates can range from 20 to 48% [4]. Once the linea alba has been incised via midline laparotomy, the healed scar tissue that results is much weaker than the uninjured fascia and can attenuate over time leading to bulge or hernia formation. The main objective of treating ventral hernias is to achieve primary fascial closure, reduce tension acting along the midline scar and add support or reinforcement to the areas of attenuated tissue. This chapter will describe the main force reduction and tissue reinforcement techniques that are the current standard of care for ventral abdominal wall reconstruction.

## 2. Primary fascial closure

One of the main determinants of abdominal wall reconstruction outcomes as it pertains to wound complication and hernia recurrence is whether the fascia can be reapproximated in the midline. While there has been some initial discussion in the literature that bridged repair may achieve similar outcomes to primary fascial closure, recent evidence clearly shows the superiority of primary fascial closure such that that every maneuver should be considered to achieve primary closure. In 2013 The MD Anderson group, published their outcomes with 222 patients who underwent either primary closure with mesh reinforcement or bridged repair. The patients undergoing bridged repairs had a significantly higher risk of hernia recurrence (56 vs. 8%), and a higher overall complication rate (74 vs. 32%). The interval to recurrence was 9-fold shorter in the bridged group [5]. A more recent study from the same group which included 535 consecutive patients with a mean follow up of 30 months reinforced the fact that primary repair had a lower hernia recurrence rate (6.2 vs. 33.3%, $p < 0.001$) and lower overall complication rate (30 vs. 59%, $p = 0.001$) than bridged repair. Propensity score analysis was used to make the comparisons less heterogeneous such that predictive factors (defect width, contamination grade and postoperative chemotherapy) that were significantly higher in the bridged hernia population and could be adjusted for to make for a stronger support of a reinforced repair rather than bridging [6]. Given the clearly demonstrated advantages of primary fascial closure, appropriate use of tension reduction techniques, which increase the likelihood of primary closure, are essential for improved outcomes in hernia reconstruction.

These tension reduction techniques take advantage of the layered anatomy of the lateral abdominal wall and can be categorized as anterior or posterior component separation, based on which layers are released.

## 3. Anterior component separation

The laterally oriented forces of the oblique muscles are translated via the rectus sheaths to the linea alba and apply tension along the midline laparotomy closure. This tension increases the risk of hernia formation and can be attenuated by disconnecting some of these components of the lateral abdominal wall. Anterior component separation was described in the 1950s but was formalized and popularized by Ramirez [7]. Ramirez and colleagues noted that the medial advancement of the external oblique muscle was restricted due to its attachments at the costal margin superiorly and the groin inferiorly. It could only be advanced by 2-cm at the epigastrium, 4-cm at the midline and 2-cm at the groin on each side. In order to be able to further medialize the rectus complex, they found it necessary to divide the external oblique fascia 2-cm lateral to the linea semilunaris from the costal margin to the inguinal ligament and then elevate the external oblique muscle off the internal oblique. Additionally, they released posterior rectus sheath. The technique avoids injury to the thoracoabdominal neurovascular bundles, which lie in the plane between the internal oblique and the transversus abdominis muscles. With this release, the rectus complex could be advanced 3-cm at the epigastrium, 5-cm in the middle and 2-cm inferiorly on each side, thereby allowing for bilateral medial migration of up to 10-cm in the midline. This technique gave surgeons the ability to achieve primary fascial closure in situations where bridged repair had been the only option. Furthermore, the repair is generally reinforced by the placement of mesh, often in the retrorectus plane [7].

The main drawback of the traditional open component release technique is the need to elevate wide soft tissue flaps that extend from the midline to 2-cm lateral to the linea semilunaris. This requires ligation of the periumbilical perforators that provide the major source of vascularity to the medial skin of the abdominal wall. Since the midline closure is subject to the highest tension, loss the periumbilical perforators can cause relative ischemia and increases the risk of soft tissue complications. Moreover, the large deadspace created by extensive undermining of the skin flaps increases the risk of seroma and abscess formation. Consequently, high rates of wound complications ranging from 24 to 50% have been reported [8, 9].

Perforator preserving techniques have, therefore, gained importance. These can be categorized into four subtypes: endoscopic component separation, open release with preservation of periumbilical perforators and surrounding soft tissue, open release with additional costal margin incisions and the MICS (Minimally Invasive Component Separation) technique. The endoscopic technique is a hybrid approach to hernia repair. The component separation portion of the procedure is performed with an endoscope but the remaining portion of the procedure is performed via an open approach. An incision is made along the anterior axillary line superiorly at the level of the costal margin or inferiorly at the level of the ASIS. Blunt dissection is then carried out to the external oblique fascia which is incised. A balloon dissector is then placed between the external oblique and internal oblique muscles and inflated to create a space. Additional ports are then placed for instrumentation and the remaining length of the external oblique fascia is divided. The endoscope is then removed and abdominal wall reconstruction with mesh placement using an open technique is performed [10].

Non-endoscopic techniques include an open technique with preservation of periumbilical perforators. In this technique, as described by Dumanian and colleagues, supraumbilical skin and fat are dissected off the anterior rectus sheath for a width of about 8 cm in order to identify the semilunar line. A second infraumbilical access to the linea semilunaris is then created by suprafascial dissection and the two spaces are connected to better visualize the linea semilunaris. Care is taken to preserve the periumbilical perforators. While this technique spares many of the periumbilical perforators, a significant amount of soft tissue undermining and elevation is performed, which increases dead space and thus the risk of wound complications [11] (**Figure 1**). Another technique by the same group uses supplemental subcostal transverse incisions through which the external oblique aponeurosis is longitudinally incised from the level of the costal margin to the inguinal ligament. This technique requires less soft tissue undermining than the previously described technique but requires transverse subcostal incisions [12].

The Minimally Invasive Component Separation (MICS) technique described by Butler et al. avoids the need for endoscopic instruments, additional access incisions and involves much less undermining and soft tissue elevation than the above described techniques. The MICS technique can be performed with either bioprosthetic as originally described [minimally invasive component separation with inlay bioprosthetic mesh (MICSIB)] or synthetic mesh placed in the retrorectus, preperitoneal or intraperitoneal plane. After the hernia has been reduced and lysis of adhesions has been completed, two horizontal subcutaneous tunnels (3-cm wide and 2-cm inferior to the costal margin) are dissected superficial to the anterior

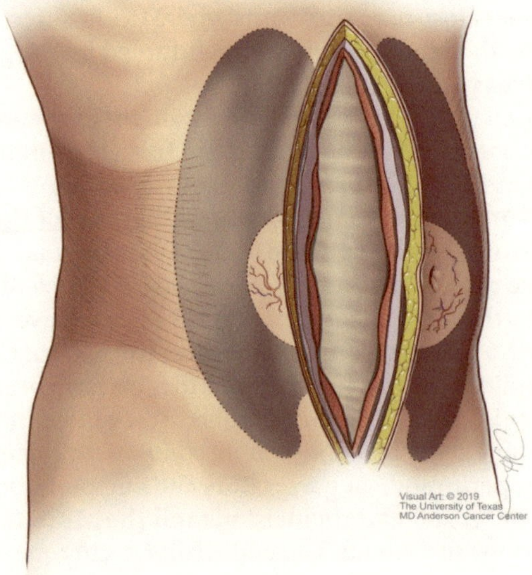


**Figure 1.**
*Area of subcutaneous dissection in periumbilical perforator sparing anterior component separation technique. Even though periumbilical perforators are spared, there is significant undermining of the subcutaneous tissue and increased risk of wound complications (Visual Art: © 2019 The University of Texas M.D. Anderson Cancer Center).*

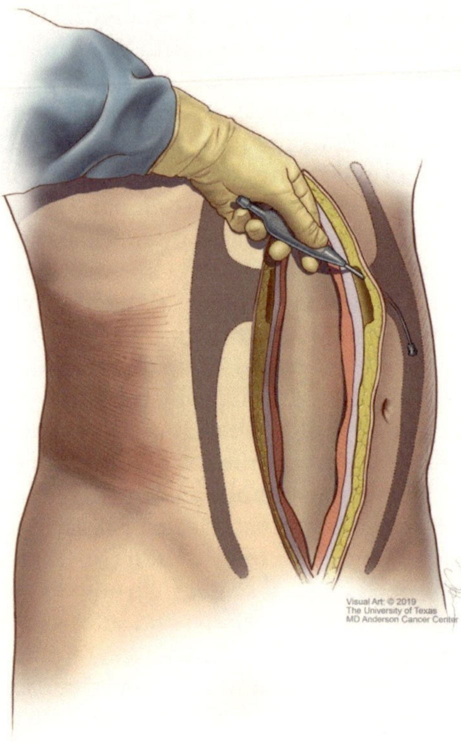


**Figure 2.**
*Area of subcutaneous dissection in the minimally invasive anterior component separation technique (MICS). Width of the horizontal and vertical tunnels is 4 and 2 cm respectively implying much less soft tissue undermining. (Visual Art: © 2019 The University of Texas M.D. Anderson Cancer Center).*

rectus sheath that extend laterally to just lateral to the linea semilunaris (**Figure 2**) Through a 2-cm long incision through the external oblique aponeurosis located 1.5 cm lateral to the linea semilunar, the Yankauer sucker is inserted and used to dissect between the internal and external oblique muscles in the loose areolar plane using sweeping motions inferiorly and superiorly. With the use of a lighted retractor, narrow vertical subcutaneous tunnels measuring 2-cm in width are dissected superficial to the external oblique aponeurosis along the path of intended aponeurotic release. With the use of Yankauer suction tip placed below the external oblique aponeurosis and pushed against the rectus complex as a guide, the external oblique fascia is incised 1.5–2-cm lateral to the linea semilunaris. Through these subcutaneous tunnels the exterior oblique aponeurosis is released from 12-cm superior to the costal margin and inferiorly to the inguinal ligament [13] (**Figure 3**).

The midline soft tissues are then elevated off the anterior sheath laterally to just medial to the medial row of rectus abdominis muscle perforators. The preperitoneal layer is dissected off the posterior rectus sheath and a bioprosthetic or synthetic mesh is placed as an underlay in the preperitoneal plane deep to the posterior rectus sheath. The mesh can also be placed in the retrorectus plane (between the rectus muscle and the posterior rectus sheath). Polypropylene sutures are used to place U-stitches between the mesh and the linea semilunaris or rectus muscle complex at least 5-cm lateral to the true fascial edge. The rectus muscle complex is primarily approximated in the midline over the mesh using interrupted or running

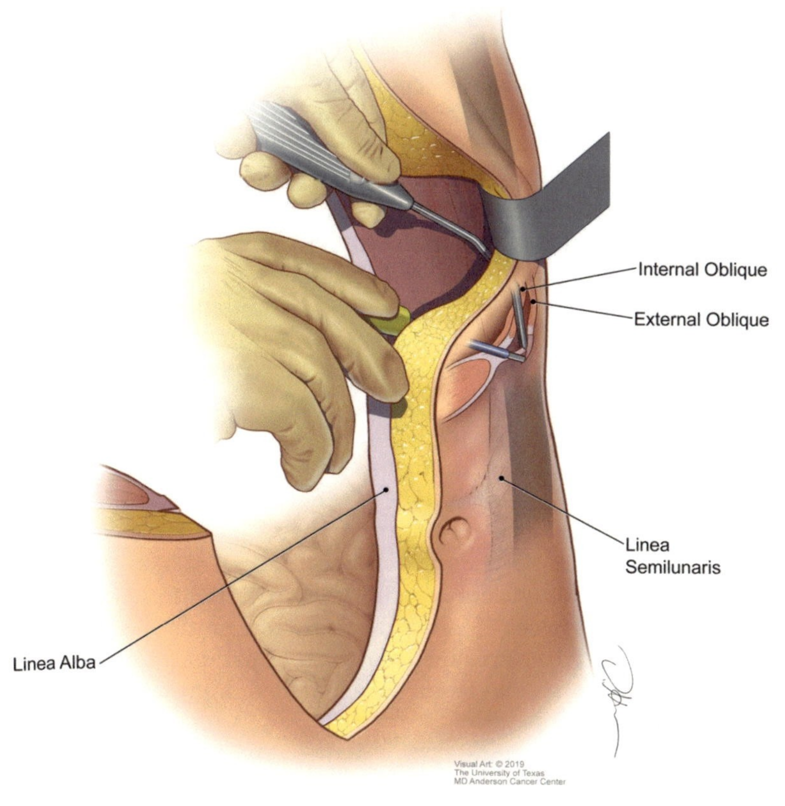


**Figure 3.**
*MICS technique demonstrating access to the external oblique fascia through a subcutaneous tunnel. The Yankauer suction tip is then used to create the plane between the external oblique and internal oblique. The external oblique fascia is then incised 1.5 cm lateral to the linea semilunaris (Visual Art: © 2019 The University of Texas M.D. Anderson Cancer Center).*

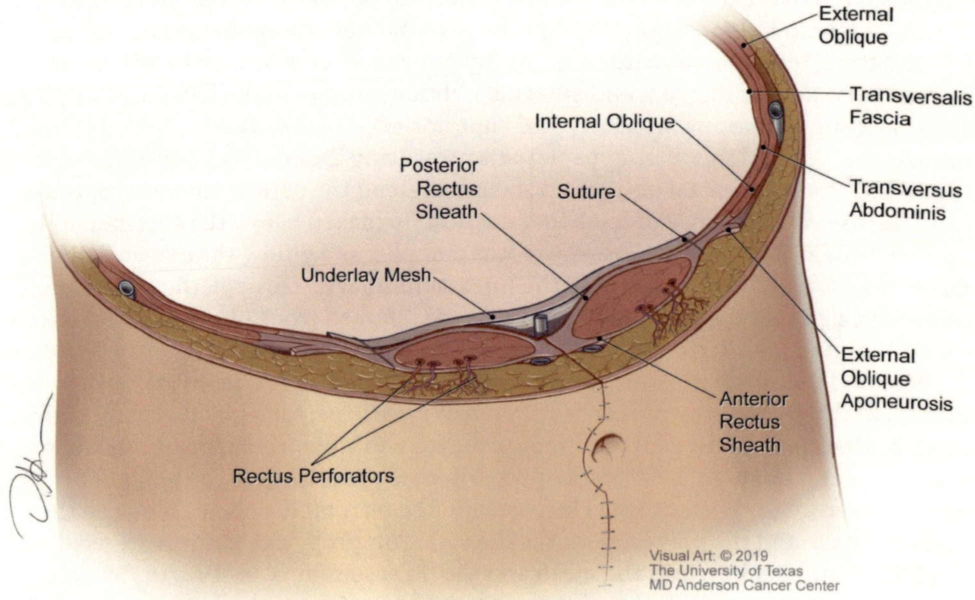


**Figure 4.**
*Cross-sectional image demonstrating release of the external oblique after anterior component separation. A mesh has been placed in the underlay plane. Rectus perforators to the overlying skin flap have been spared (Visual Art: © 2019 The University of Texas M.D. Anderson Cancer Center).*

#1 polypropylene sutures. Deadspace reduction is achieved by placing resorbable quilting sutures between the posterior sheath and the mesh as well as between the anterior rectus sheath and the overlying elevated soft tissue. Drains are placed between the underlay mesh and the fascial closure, the component separation donor sites and in the subcutaneous plane along the midline closure (**Figure 4**).

As expected, these modifications to the traditional open technique improve vascularity to the overlying soft tissue, reduce deadspace and significantly decrease wound complications. A review of 107 patients who underwent abdominal wall reconstruction using either an open technique or the MICS technique showed that, despite a larger mean hernia defect size, patients undergoing the MICS technique had a significantly lower rate of skin dehiscence (11 vs. 28%; $p < 0.011$), and wound healing complications (14 vs. 32%; $p < 0.026$) [14].

While anterior component separation has multiple advantages, some surgeons raised concerns about using this technique in the setting of rectus muscle violation. The main concern was that prior injury to the rectus muscle complex due to direct incision or excision of the muscle or due to placement of an ostomy or tube through it would increase the risk of scarring and prevent safe component release and adequate medial migration [15]. In order to further study this issue, the MD Anderson group performed a retrospective review of patients with or without prior rectus muscle violation, who underwent subsequent abdominal wall reconstruction using anterior component separation, was conducted. A total of 68% of patients in the study had rectus violation while 32% of patients did not. Patients in the rectus violation group had elevated BMI, larger hernia defects, increased incidence of chemotherapy and two or more prior operations. Yet, the overall wound healing, hernia recurrence and complication rates were similar in the 2 groups. The study also noted that the type of rectus violation (prior incision/excision of muscle or ostomy/tube placement) did not influence complication rates [16]. Anterior component separation remains a safe and effective technique even in the setting of prior or concurrent rectus violation.

## 4. Posterior component separation

In addition to anterior component separation, posterior releases of the abdominal musculofascial components have been described. Posterior component separation (PCS) such as the transverse abdominis muscle release (TAR), have evolved as extensions of the Rives-Stoppa repair. The Rives-Stoppa repair, described in the 1970s, involves elevation of the posterior rectus sheath in the retrorectus plane laterally to the linea semilunaris [17]. While the traditional repair stops here, the TAR technique involves division of the transversus abdominis muscle followed by dissection laterally between the transversus abdominis muscle and the transversalis fascia followed by wide mesh reinforcement [18]. Once the thoracolumbar intercostal nerves are visualized along the lateral edge of the rectus muscle complex, the posterior lamella of the internal oblique muscle is incised medial to these nerves which exposes the transversus abdominis muscle. The transversus muscle is then incised to reach the plane between the transversus abdominis muscle and transversalis fascia (**Figure 5**). This plane of dissection can be extended laterally to the psoas muscles thereby allowing for placement of a very large mesh (**Figures 6** and 7). Proponents of this technique claim that it can provide up to 10-cm of medialization of the rectus muscle complex and have demonstrated promising outcomes [19]. A retrospective review of 428 patients who

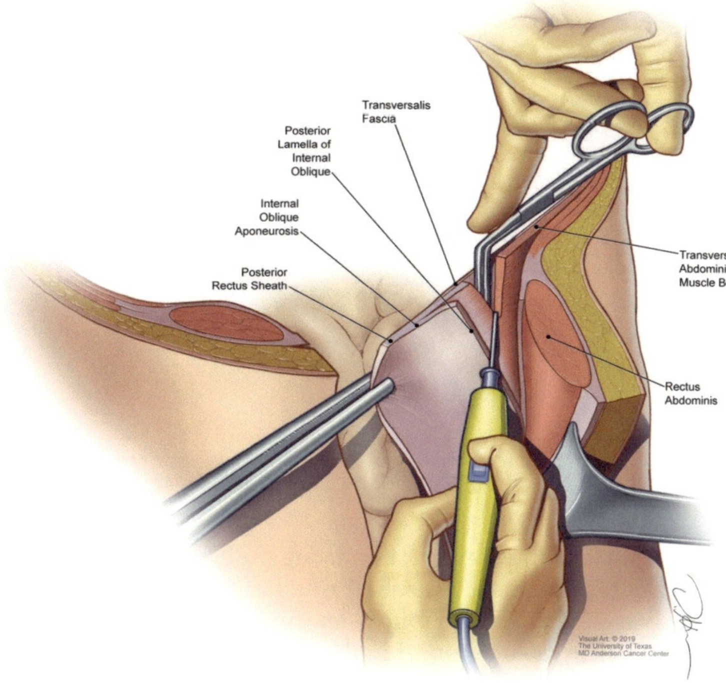


**Figure 5.**
*Transversus abdominis release technique demonstrating that the posterior lamella of the internal oblique aponeurosis has been incised to provide access to the transversus abdominis muscle. The transversus abdominis muscle is then incised. The plane between the internal oblique and transversus abdominis muscle is not opened or disturbed (Visual Art: © 2019 The University of Texas M.D. Anderson Cancer Center).*

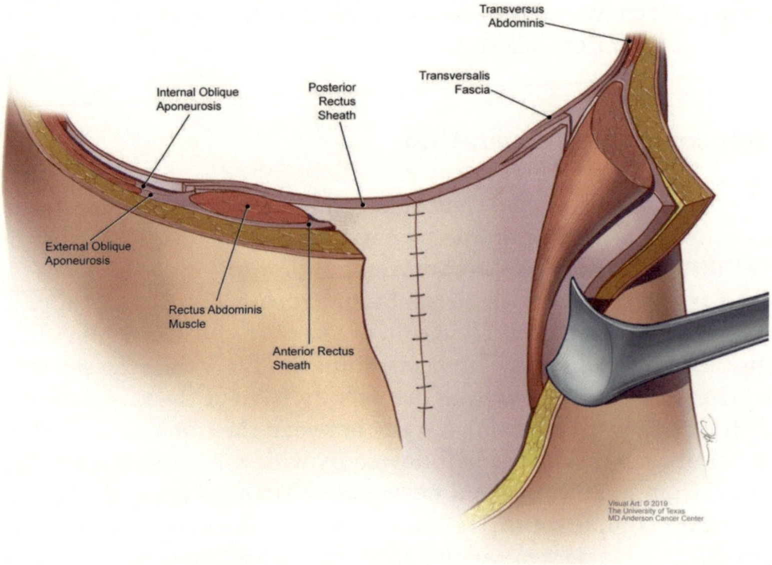


**Figure 6.**
*Posterior sheath is approximated following transversus abdominis muscle release.*

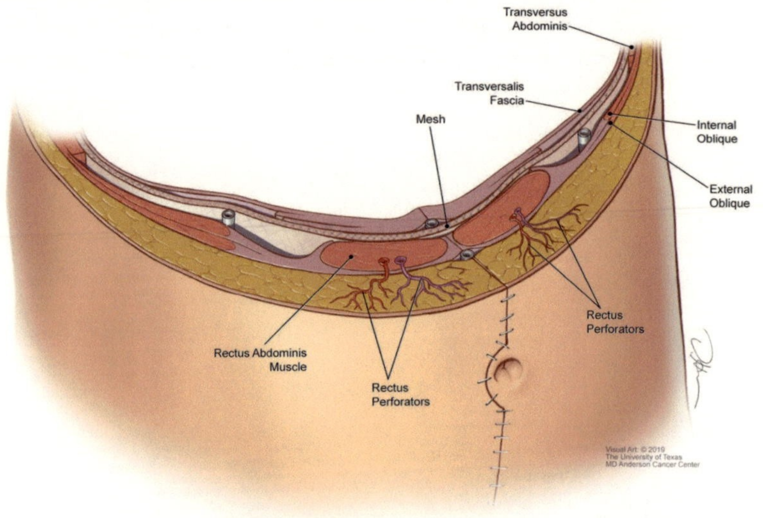


**Figure 7.**
*Cross-sectional image demonstrating Transversus abdominis release (posterior component separation) with retrorectus placement of mesh (Visual Art: © 2019 The University of Texas M.D. Anderson Cancer Center).*

underwent abdominal wall reconstruction using the TAR technique were noted to have a surgical site occurrence rate of 18% and a 30 day SSI of 9.1%. Hernia recurrence rate was 3.7% at a mean follow-up time of 31.5 months, which is lower than average recurrence rates reported in the literature [20]. Since the TAR release is always accompanied by a very wide mesh, it is unclear if the benefits of lower hernia recurrence are related to the reduction in tension by the TAR release or the extra wide placement of mesh. One benefit of the TAR includes being able to place a large mesh in the pretransversalis fascial plane so there is essentially no risk of bowel exposure to mesh. Another major benefit is that skin flaps do not have to be elevated thus reducing the risk of medical skin ischemia. The TAR release is considered the dominant posterior component release technique and is sometimes referred to as posterior component separation in the literature (PCS).

While both anterior and posterior component separation techniques are commonly used for abdominal wall reconstruction there have been few head to head comparisons between the techniques. Useful comparative analysis is difficult given the heterogeneity of hernia defects and the biases related to surgeon preferences and patient selection. In 2012 Krpata and colleagues published a retrospective review comparing outcomes following anterior component separation (ACS) and transversus abdominis muscle release (TAR) in their patient population. They found that the overall complication rate was significantly lower for TAR (25.5%) compared to ACS (48.2%) and also noted a higher hernia recurrence rate for ACS (14.3%) vs. TAR (3.6%), but this was not statistically significant [21]. The ACS repairs in this study were performed using traditional open techniques, which as described earlier, are known to have a higher rate of wound healing complications than the more recent perforator sparing techniques. Furthermore, 38% of patients undergoing ACS underwent simultaneous panniculectomy compared to 4% of TAR patients which could bias the complication profile in favor of TAR. It is not unreasonable to believe that higher wound complication rates would translate to increased risk of hernia recurrence. A more recent study published in 2017 that compared MICS to posterior component separation noted a much lower rate of complications for the ACS repairs and no significant difference in complication profile or recurrence rates between TAR and anterior MICS [22]. They did note that a slightly higher hernia recurrence risk with the MICS technique but this was not statistically different. Based on their description they did not release superior to the costal margin. The full benefit of the MICS release is attained when the release is extended 12-cm superior to the costal margin, especially when treating epigastric hernias. Large prospective studies are needed to better compare these techniques, however both anterior and posterior components are widely practiced by surgeons. Choice between the techniques generally depends on surgeon preference and training [23].

## 5. Mesh types and plane of mesh placement

In addition to tension reduction techniques, the use of mesh reinforcement has significantly improved hernia recurrence rates. Previous landmark studies demonstrated that when mesh was used for the repair hernia recurrence rate was reduced my almost 50% compared to fascial closure alone at three and 10 year follow up [24, 25]. Synthetic and bioprosthetic mesh are the two major categories of mesh in use today. Polypropylene, polyester and polytetrafluoroethylene (PTFE) are common polymers used to create synthetic mesh material. Multiple studies over the past two decades have been performed in order to identify the clinically relevant features of different mesh architectures [26]. In general, these mesh materials can vary with respect to their pore-size and weight. Studies have shown that lighter weight mesh materials with large pore sizes induce increased type 1 collagen deposition and demonstrate an increase in tensile strength over time. They demonstrate better incorporation and improved abdominal wall compliance compared to mesh with smaller pore sizes [27]. Light weight mesh materials, however, have an increased risk of mesh fracture. Small pore sizes increase the risk of bridging fibrosis and rigid scar formation which reduces the compliance of the reinforced abdominal wall [28]. PTFE has the smallest pores size which reduces adhesion formation, however, since the pore size is too small for macrophages to enter, the clearance of bacteria and/or biofilm is very difficult and the mesh usually needs to be explanted in the setting of persistent infection [29]. Ideally synthetic meshes need to be created using strong, yet complaint materials that do not induce visceral adhesion formation.

A newer subtype of synthetic meshes consisting of resorbable materials, such as polyglycolic acid (PGA), polylactic acid (PLA), trimethyl carbonate (TMC) and poly-4-hydroxybuturate (P4HB), has been recently introduced. Each of these materials varies in the absorption rates and mechanisms and can be combined to develop mesh with different profiles. The main proposed advantage is that these materials can resorb and therefore have less associated long-term foreign body reaction, lower risk of infection and preserved compliance [30]. There have been few outcomes-based studies with these mesh materials with regard to long-term recurrence rates. The Complex Open Bioresorbable Reconstruction of the Abdominal Wall (COBRA) Study analyzed outcomes related to PGA/TMC absorbable mesh and reported 28% SSO and 18% SSI rates. Recurrence rate was 17% at 2 years. More in depth studies and comparative analysis are necessary before these materials can be universally adopted [31]. The indications for these materials are not yet clear.

Synthetic meshes, although very reasonably priced, are associated with an increased risk of adhesion or fistula formation if placed in contact with abdominal viscera and an increased risk of infection when placed in contaminated wounds. Bioprosthetic meshes were introduced to mitigate some of these drawbacks related to infection and adhesion formation. Bioprosthetic meshes are generally derived from human, porcine or bovine sources and mainly consist of dermis, pericardium or intestinal submucosa. Acellular dermal matrix (ADM) is the most common substrate used in abdominal wall reinforcement [32]. Radiation and chemical or enzymatic treatment are used to decellularize, sterilize and treat the matrix to reduce the likelihood of a host rejection response. These processes are not benign and may alter the characteristics of the mesh and reduce its potential to integrate with the surrounding tissues. Increased cross-linking, caused by some of these treatments, inhibits tissue and vascular ingrowth and integration, which lead to scarring or encapsulation as seen with synthetic meshes [33]. This phenomenon was witnessed when a highly cross-linked porcine acellular dermal matrix (Permacol; Medtronic, Minneapolis, MN) was compared to a non-cross linked matrix (Strattice; LifeCell Corp. Branchburg, NJ). The study showed that while the two meshes did not differ with respect to the hernia or bulge recurrence, there was a significantly higher risk SSI associated with the cross linked mesh [34].

The mesh types can also be affected by the source from which the tissue was harvested. For instance, compared to xenogeneic mesh, human dermal matrix has a higher proportion of elastin and a faster remodeling rate [35]. Therefore, bioprosthetic meshes harvested from human skin have higher hernia and bulge occurrence. While this feature might be useful in other indications for soft tissue support, such as breast reconstruction, it is disadvantageous in abdominal wall reconstructions and has been mostly abandoned by hernia surgeons [36]. Comparison between bovine and porcine derived meshes however have not yielded significant long-term differences with respect to hernia recurrence or SSOs [37, 38].

While large long-term, head to head comparisons between synthetic and bioprosthetic mesh products have been lacking, there have been multiple studies with each of these products. Carbonell and colleagues conducted a retrospective review of 100 patients who underwent ventral hernia repair with macroporous light-weight synthetic mesh in clean-contaminated (42 patients) and a contaminated (58 patients) setting and were followed only for a mean of 10.8 months. They reported a 7% SSI rate, 31% SSO rate and a 7% recurrence rate. They also had a 4%

mesh explantation rate [39]. The experience with bioprosthetic meshes has been variable [40]. The MD Anderson group compared outcomes using bioprosthetic mesh in clean (CDC Class 1) vs. combined contaminated [clean-contaminated (Class 2) + Contaminated (Class 3) + Dirty/Infected (Class 4)] cases in a review of 359 patients followed for a much longer mean follow-up of 28 months. The analysis demonstrated no significant difference in overall 30 day SSI, hernia recurrence rates or mesh removal rates in the clean vs. combined contaminated groups. Factors independently predictive of hernia recurrence included bridged repair, use of human ADM, reoperation and mesh removal. The study demonstrated increasing wound related SSOs with increasing CDC classification however the wounds did not progress to higher overall SSI or recurrent hernia rates [41]. A more recent study using propensity score matched groups on a similar group of patients from the same institution demonstrated even more compelling results. In this study of 519 patients, 420 patients underwent abdominal wall reconstruction with bioprosthetic mesh placement in ventral hernia working group (VHWG) Class 1 or 2 wounds and 99 patients underwent mesh placement in Class 3 and 4 wounds. No differences were seen in wound related outcomes, infections, dehiscences, reoperation and hernia recurrence [42]. Consequently the VHWG promotes the use of bioprosthetic meshes in grade 3 or 4 cases [43].

The plane of mesh placement is another important factor that may affect outcomes. An ideal plane for mesh placement should be deep enough to reduce susceptibility to superficial skin and soft tissue infection or cutaneous exposure in the event of skin separation. Contact with bowel or intraperitoneal contents should be avoided in order to reduce the risk of bowel adhesion and possible enterocutaneous fistula formation. Antiadhesive, barrier-coated meshes have been used to reduce intestinal adhesions associated with intraperitoneal macroporous synthetic mesh placement [44]. Recent analyses have also shown that SSI and hernia recurrence is much higher in mesh placed as onlay (superficial to the fascial closure), or interposition configurations (bridged repair without fascial closure), than when mesh has been placed in sublay fashion (retrorectus, intraperitoneal or preperitoneal plane). These findings have been noted in laparoscopic as well as open repairs [45].

## 6. Soft tissue coverage options

Successful reconstruction of the abdominal wall relies on robust well vascularized overlying soft tissue. The main drawback of the traditional anterior component technique was related to poor vascularization of the overlying skin flaps caused by the disruption of the rectus abdominis perforators. In many scenarios the overlying soft tissues may be compromised due to massive ventral hernia, prior trauma, surgical incisions or tumor resection. In addition to restoring the myofascial integrity using tension reducing component separation techniques and mesh reinforcement of the abdominal wall, it may be necessary to take additional steps to restore the overlying soft tissue [46].

Options for soft tissue coverage in the case of skin deficiency depend upon surface area and location of the defect and may involve the use of local tissue rearrangement, pedicled flaps or free flaps. From the standpoint of soft tissue reconstruction, defects can be characterized as epigastric, periumbilical, hypogastric or suprapubic defects. Small defects in all locations can be reconstructed with local advancement or rotational advancement of tissue based upon available soft tissue laxity.

However, intermediate to large size defects may require more extensive techniques for soft tissue transfer. Superior skin defects located laterally may be reconstructed using pedicled flaps based on the thoracodorsal or circumflex scapular vascular pedicles. These include latissimus dorsi flaps, serratus or parascapular flaps. These reconstructions require an intraoperative position change, which may increase operative time. In certain cases, when the defect lies beyond the reach of a pedicled flap, a free tissue transfer often with the use of interposition vein grafts is necessary [47, 48].

For midline skin defect between the xiphoid and umbilicus, there are no reliable pedicled flap options. These defects usually need to be reconstructed with a free flap from the thigh or back, often with vein grafts. Inferior, medial and lateral skin defects can usually be reconstructed using pedicled thigh-based flaps. These include pedicled anterolateral thigh flaps, rectus femoris or subtotal thigh flaps. It is best to use mesh to reconstruct the musculofascial component of a composite (soft tissue and musculofascial) defect rather than the fascia from a fasciocutaneous flap. The flap fascia is unreliable and associated with increased risk of hernia and bulge [47, 49]. For defects that are too large or out of reach of pedicled flaps, free flaps need to be used. In addition to the complexity associated with free tissue transfer, the lack of useful local recipient vessels is a significant hurdle. It is generally important to avoid the use of intraperitoneal recipient vessels. An iatrogenic hernia must be created to allow the pedicle to traverse the mesh-musculofascial reconstruction which can result in a pedicle kink leading to flap vascular compromise and/or symptomatic hernia formation. In addition, the management of flap vascular compromise requires a reoperative laparotomy to access the anastomosis. The main recipient vessels include the internal mammary, inferior epigastric, axillary and femoral vessels. If the free flap pedicle is too short, cephalic or saphenous vein grafts are used as interposition graft between the flap pedicle and the recipient vessels. In many cases an arteriovenous vein loop is created by anastomosing the saphenous vein to the superficial femoral artery and then transferred to the abdomen to serve as a useful recipient. Healthy soft tissue coverage reduces risk of infection, helps reduce the effect of radiation, increases likelihood of mesh integration and therefore contributes to lower incidence of soft tissue complications and hernia recurrence [47, 50].

Excess subcutaneous tissue, on the other hand, can cause increased physical strain on wound closures and heighten the risk of dehiscence. In these situations, the redundant tissue should be addressed using a panniculectomy. Use of a panniculectomy in the setting of ventral hernia repair has been associated with higher wound morbidity, increased rates of fat necrosis and abscess formation but similar overall complication and hernia recurrence rates to abdominal reconstruction without panniculectomy [51]. Vertical excess can be removed via an elliptical or tear drop incision. Simultaneous horizontal and vertical excess can be removed using a combined longitudinal and transverse panniculectomy in a fleur-de-lis pattern. Due to an increase in wound breakdown at the central trifurcation point of this incision, Butler and Reis described a modified "mercedes" incision pattern. The shorter triangle flaps with a more obtuse angle at the trifurcation or T-junction and the more cephalad location of this trifurcation point reduces the risk of breakdown by improving blood flow and relocating the trifurcation point further away from the groin and appearing like a "Mercedes" symbol [52].

The use of closed incision negative pressure wound therapy has also improved wound related outcomes in high risk patients. Negative pressure wound therapy has yielded statistically lower wound complications and surgical site occurrences [53]. Further modifications of this technique such as partial closure of the incision and management of both open and closed areas with negative pressure therapy, described as the "French Fry or String of pearls" technique are also gaining interest [54].

## 7. Preoperative optimization

There are multiple intraoperative techniques that have improved outcomes in ventral hernia reconstruction, however when possible, every attempt should be made to optimize the patient prior to surgery. This can be achieved my managing or alleviating certain modifiable risk factors that have been shown to increase the risk of complications and include smoking, diabetes control, and obesity [55].

Smoking has been shown to increase risk of hypoperfusion, especially to the undermined flap, and lead to tissue necrosis and abscess formation. In a systematic review of 6 randomized trials and 15 observational studies, the authors found that each week of smoking cessation increases the magnitude of effect by 19%. Trials of 4 weeks of smoking cessation had a significantly larger effect than shorter trials [56]. Nicotine replacement therapy, however, has not been shown to have a detrimental impact to wound healing and complications in gastrointestinal surgery [57].

Diabetes control in the perioperative setting is another important factor in reducing risk of infection and complications. Postoperative hyperglycemia >200 and a Hemoglobin A1c greater than 6.5 have been associated with a 3-fold higher rate of wound dehiscence in certain studies. Perioperative blood glucose should be maintained below 120–160 mg/dl. Even a single instance of postoperative hyperglycemia greater than 200 mg/dl has been shown to significantly increase dehiscence risk [58–60].

Obesity is well known factor that has been shown to increase the risk of SSO following ventral hernia repair. A study published in 2016 reviewed 313 patients who underwent complex hernia repair analyzed the effect of obesity over a 15.6 month follow-up. They divided the population based on BMI according the World Health Organization (WHO) classification and found a significantly higher risk of hernia recurrence and reoperation in patients with increasing BMI [61]. Contrary to this, a more recent larger study from the MD Anderson group including 511 patients with a longer mean follow-up of 32 months demonstrated that class 1 or higher obesity does not affect hernia recurrence rates. Increasing class of obesity, however, does increase the risk of SSOs such as infection, fat necrosis, skin dehiscence [62]. An inflection point above which SSO became a considerable problem was noted to be a BMI of 31.9. It is important to understand that most patients in this study had a BMI less than 40. Hernia recurrence has been shown to increase as the BMI increases over 40. (2-year recurrence rate 8% of BMI between 30 and 39 which then increases to 25% for BMI between 40 and 49 and 45% in patients with BMI > 50) [55].

## 8. Conclusion

Abdominal wall reconstruction has multiple complex nuances which need to be understood and adjusted based on the clinical scenario. In order to improve outcomes, the patient needs to be optimized from the standpoint of modifiable risk factors such as diabetes, obesity and tobacco use. Next, procedures to reduce tension and achieve primary closure such as anterior and posterior component separation need to be performed. Anterior component separation has been associated with wound related complications which can be prevented by minimally invasive techniques designed to spare perforators as described in this chapter.

The repair then needs to be reinforced with synthetic or biologic mesh. Bioprosthetic mesh has been shown to have a low rate of surgical site complications in contaminated cases. Finally, techniques of maintaining well perfused soft tissue coverage is important and can be achieved by local rearrangement of tissue, pedicled flaps or free flaps. All of these factors, including clinical features of the case, and surgeon familiarity with the technique help facilitate a successful outcome.

## Author details

Sahil K. Kapur and Charles E. Butler*
Department of Plastic Surgery, The University of Texas MD Anderson Cancer Center, Houston, TX, United States

*Address all correspondence to: cbutler@mdanderson.org

## References

[1] Pollock AV, Evans M. Early prediction of late incisional hernias. British Journal of Surgery. 1989;**76**(9):953-954

[2] Cobb WS, Kercher KW, Heniford BT. Laparoscopic repair of incisional hernia. Surgical Clinics. 2005;**85**(1):91-103

[3] Israelsson LA, Jonsson T. Incisional hernia after midline laparotomy: A prospective study. The European Journal of Surgery. 1996;**162**(2):125-129

[4] Poulose BK, Shelton J, Phillips S, Moore D, Nealon W, Penson D, et al. Epidemiology and cost of ventral hernia repair: Making the case for hernia research. Hernia. 2012;**16**(2):179-183

[5] Booth JH, Garvey PB, Baumann DP, Selber JC, Nguyen AT, Clemens MW, et al. Primary fascial closure with mesh reinforcement is superior to bridged mesh repair for abdominal wall reconstruction. Journal of the American College of Surgeons. 2013;**217**(6):999-1009

[6] Giordano S, Garvey PB, Baumann DP, Liu J, Butler CE. Primary fascial closure with biologic mesh reinforcement results in lesser complication and recurrence rates than bridged biologic mesh repair for abdominal wall reconstruction: A propensity score analysis. Surgery. 2017;**161**(2):499-508

[7] Ramirez OM, Ruas E, Dellon AL. "Components separation" method for closure of abdominal-wall defects: An anatomic and clinical study. Plastic and Reconstructive Surgery. 1990;**86**(3):519-526

[8] de Vries Reilingh TS, van Goor H, Charbon JA, Rosman C, Hesselink EJ, van der Wilt G-J, et al. Repair of giant midline abdominal wall hernias: "components separation technique" versus prosthetic repair. World Journal of Surgery. 2007;**31**(4):756-763

[9] de Vries RT, Bodegom M, Van Goor H, Hartman E, van der Wilt GJ, Bleichrodt R. Autologous tissue repair of large abdominal wall defects. British Journal of Surgery. 2007;**94**(7):791-803

[10] Giurgius M, Bendure L, Davenport DL, Roth JS. The endoscopic component separation technique for hernia repair results in reduced morbidity compared to the open component separation technique. Hernia. 2012;**16**(1):47-51

[11] Saulis AS, Dumanian GA. Periumbilical rectus abdominis perforator preservation significantly reduces superficial wound complications in "separation of parts" hernia repairs. Plastic and Reconstructive Surgery. 2002;**109**(7):2275-2280

[12] Dumanian GA. Abdominal wall reconstruction. In: Grabb and Smith's Plastic Surgery: Seventh Edition. Wolters Kluwer Health Adis (ESP). Philadelphia, PA, USA: Lippincott Williams & Wilkins; 2013. pp. 933-940

[13] Butler CE, Campbell KT. Minimally invasive component separation with inlay bioprosthetic mesh (MICSIB) for complex abdominal wall reconstruction. Plastic and Reconstructive Surgery. 2011;**128**(3):698-709

[14] Ghali S, Turza KC, Baumann DP, Butler CE. Minimally invasive component separation results in fewer wound-healing complications than open component separation for large ventral hernia repairs. Journal of the American College of Surgeons. 2012;**214**(6):981-989

[15] Lowe JB, Garza JR, Bowman JL, Rohrich RJ, Strodel W. Endoscopically

assisted "components separation" for closure of abdominal wall defects. Plastic and Reconstructive Surgery. 2000;**105**(2):720-730

[16] Garvey PB, Bailey CM, Baumann DP, Liu J, Butler CE. Violation of the rectus complex is not a contraindication to component separation for abdominal wall reconstruction. Journal of the American College of Surgeons. 2012;**214**(2):131-139

[17] Stoppa RE. The treatment of complicated groin and incisional hernias. World Journal of Surgery. 1989;**13**(5):545-554

[18] Novitsky YW, Elliott HL, Orenstein SB, Rosen MJ. Transversus abdominis muscle release: A novel approach to posterior component separation during complex abdominal wall reconstruction. American Journal of Surgery. 2012;**204**(5):709-716

[19] Majumder A, Miller H, Del Campo L, Soltanian H, Novitsky Y. Assessment of myofascial medialization following posterior component separation via transversus abdominis muscle release in a cadaveric model. Hernia. 2018;**22**:637-644

[20] Novitsky YW, Fayezizadeh M, Majumder A, Neupane R, Elliott HL, Orenstein SB. Outcomes of posterior component separation with transversus abdominis muscle release and synthetic mesh sublay reinforcement. Annals of Surgery. 2016;**264**(2):226-232

[21] Krpata DM, Blatnik JA, Novitsky YW, Rosen MJ. Posterior and open anterior components separations: A comparative analysis. American Journal of Surgery. 2012;**203**(3):318-322

[22] Parent B, Horn D, Jacobson L, Petersen RP, Hinojosa M, Yates R, et al. Wound morbidity in minimally invasive anterior component separation compared to transversus abdominis release. Plastic and Reconstructive Surgery. 2017;**139**(2):472-479

[23] Kumar S, Edmunds RW, Dowdy C, Chang Y-WW, King R, Roth JS. Anterior versus posterior component separation: Which is better? Plastic and Reconstructive Surgery. 2018;**142**(3S):47S-53S

[24] Luijendijk RW, Hop WC, Van Den Tol MP, De Lange DC, Braaksma MM, IJzermans JN, et al. A comparison of suture repair with mesh repair for incisional hernia. New England Journal of Medicine. 2000;**343**(6):392-398

[25] Burger JW, Luijendijk RW, Hop WC, Halm JA, Verdaasdonk EG, Jeekel J. Long-term follow-up of a randomized controlled trial of suture versus mesh repair of incisional hernia. Annals of Surgery. 2004;**240**(4):578

[26] Cobb WS. A current review of synthetic meshes in abdominal wall reconstruction. Plastic and Reconstructive Surgery. 2018;**142**(3S):64S-71S

[27] Greca F, Paula J, Biondo-Simões M, Costa F, Silva A, Time S, et al. The influence of differing pore sizes on the biocompatibility of two polypropylene meshes in the repair of abdominal defects. Hernia. 2001;**5**(2):59-64

[28] Cobb WS, Warren JA, Ewing JA, Burnikel A, Merchant M, Carbonell AM. Open retromuscular mesh repair of complex incisional hernia: Predictors of wound events and recurrence. Journal of the American College of Surgeons. 2015;**220**(4):606-613

[29] Hawn MT, Gray SH, Snyder CW, Graham LA, Finan KR, Vick CC. Predictors of mesh explantation after incisional hernia repair. The American Journal of Surgery. 2011;**202**(1):28-33

[30] Kim M, Oommen B, Ross S, Lincourt A, Matthews B, Heniford B, et al. The current status of biosynthetic mesh for ventral hernia repair. Surgical Technology International. 2014;**25**:114-121

[31] Rosen MJ, Bauer JJ, Harmaty M, Carbonell AM, Cobb WS, Matthews B, et al. Multicenter, prospective, longitudinal study of the recurrence, surgical site infection, and quality of life after contaminated ventral hernia repair using biosynthetic absorbable mesh: The COBRA study. Annals of Surgery. 2017;**265**(1):205

[32] Nahabedian MY, Sosin M, Bhanot P. A current review of biologic meshes in abdominal wall reconstruction. Plastic and Reconstructive Surgery. 2018;**142**(3S):74S-81S

[33] Butler CE, Burns NK, Campbell KT, Mathur AB, Jaffari MV, Rios CN. Comparison of cross-linked and non-cross-linked porcine acellular dermal matrices for ventral hernia repair. Journal of the American College of Surgeons. 2010;**211**(3):368-376

[34] Cheng AW, Abbas MA, Tejirian T. Outcome of abdominal wall hernia repair with biologic mesh: Permacol™ versus Strattice™. The American Surgeon. 2014;**80**(10):999-1002

[35] Campbell KT, Burns NK, Rios CN, Mathur AB, Butler CE. Human versus non-cross-linked porcine acellular dermal matrix used for ventral hernia repair: Comparison of in vivo fibrovascular remodeling and mechanical repair strength. Plastic and Reconstructive Surgery. 2011;**127**(6):2321-2332

[36] Bluebond-Langner R, Keifa ES, Mithani S, Bochicchio GV, Scalea T, Rodriguez ED. Recurrent abdominal laxity following interpositional human acellular dermal matrix. Annals of Plastic Surgery. 2008;**60**(1):76-80

[37] Clemens M, Selber J, Adelman D, Baumann D, Garvey P, Butler C. Bovine versus porcine acellular dermal matrix for complex abdominal wall reconstruction. Plastic and Reconstructive Surgery. 2012;**130**(1S):64

[38] Clemens MW, Selber JC, Liu J, Adelman DM, Baumann DP, Garvey PB, et al. Bovine versus porcine acellular dermal matrix for complex abdominal wall reconstruction. Plastic and Reconstructive Surgery. 2013;**131**(1):71-79

[39] Carbonell AM, Criss CN, Cobb WS, Novitsky YW, Rosen MJ. Outcomes of synthetic mesh in contaminated ventral hernia repairs. Journal of the American College of Surgeons. 2013;**217**(6):991-998

[40] Itani KM, Rosen M, Vargo D, Awad SS, Denoto G 3rd, Butler CE, et al. Prospective study of single-stage repair of contaminated hernias using a biologic porcine tissue matrix: The RICH study. Surgery. 2012;**152**(3):498-505

[41] Garvey PB, Martinez RA, Baumann DP, Liu J, Butler CE. Outcomes of abdominal wall reconstruction with acellular dermal matrix are not affected by wound contamination. Journal of the American College of Surgeons. 2014;**219**(5):853-864

[42] Giordano S, Largo R, Garvey PB, Baumann DP, Liu J, Butler CE. Wound contamination does not affect outcomes with acellular dermal matrix in abdominal wall reconstruction: Evidence from propensity score analysis. Plastic and Reconstructive Surgery. Global Open. 2016; **4**(9 Suppl):115

[43] Breuing K, Butler CE, Ferzoco S, Franz M, Hultman CS, Kilbridge JF, et al. Incisional ventral hernias: Review

of the literature and recommendations regarding the grading and technique of repair. Surgery. 2010;**148**(3):544-558

[44] Schreinemacher MH, van Barneveld KW, Dikmans RE, Gijbels MJ, Greve JW, Bouvy ND. Coated meshes for hernia repair provide comparable intraperitoneal adhesion prevention. Surgical Endoscopy. 2013;**27**(11):4202-4209

[45] Sosin M, Nahabedian MY, Bhanot P. The perfect plane: A systematic review of mesh location and outcomes, update 2018. Plastic and Reconstructive Surgery. 2018;**142**(3S):107S-116S

[46] Khansa I, Janis JE. Complex open abdominal wall reconstruction: Management of the skin and subcutaneous tissue. Plastic and Reconstructive Surgery. 2018;**142**(3S):125S-132S

[47] Baumann DP, Butler CE. Flap reconstruction of the abdominal wall. In: Hernia Surgery. Switzerland: Springer, Springer International Publishing; 2016. pp. 313-321

[48] Mericli AF, Garvey PB, Giordano S, Liu J, Baumann DP, Butler CE. Abdominal wall reconstruction with concomitant ostomy-associated hernia repair: Outcomes and propensity score analysis. Journal of the American College of Surgeons. 2017;**224**(3): 351-361 e2

[49] Lin SJ, Butler CE. Subtotal thigh flap and bioprosthetic mesh reconstruction for large, composite abdominal wall defects. Plastic and Reconstructive Surgery. 2010;**125**(4):1146-1156

[50] Mericli AF, Baumann DP, Butler CE. Reconstruction of the abdominal wall after oncologic resection: Defect classification and management strategies. Plastic and Reconstructive Surgery. 2018;**142**(3S):187S-196S

[51] Giordano S, Garvey PB, Baumann DP, Liu J, Butler CE. Concomitant panniculectomy affects wound morbidity but not hernia recurrence rates in abdominal wall reconstruction: A propensity score analysis. Plastic and Reconstructive Surgery. 2017;**140**(6):1263-1273

[52] Butler CE, Reis SM. Mercedes panniculectomy with simultaneous component separation ventral hernia repair. Plastic and Reconstructive Surgery. 2010;**125**(3):94e-98e

[53] Condé-Green A, Chung TL, Holton LH III, Hui-Chou HG, Zhu Y, Wang H, et al. Incisional negative-pressure wound therapy versus conventional dressings following abdominal wall reconstruction: A comparative study. Annals of Plastic Surgery. 2013;**71**(4):394-397

[54] Chopra K, Tadisina KK, Singh DP. The 'French Fry'VAC technique: Hybridisation of traditional open wound NPWT with closed incision NPWT. International Wound Journal. 2016;**13**(2):216-219

[55] Joslyn NA, Esmonde NO, Martindale RG, Hansen J, Khansa I, Janis JE. Evidence-based strategies for the Prehabilitation of the Abdominal Wall reconstruction patient. Plastic and Reconstructive Surgery. 2018;**142**(3S):21S-29S

[56] Mills E, Eyawo O, Lockhart I, Kelly S, Wu P, Ebbert JO. Smoking cessation reduces postoperative complications: A systematic review and meta-analysis. The American Journal of Medicine. 2011;**124**(2):144-154 e8

[57] Lindström D, Azodi OS, Wladis A, Tønnesen H, Linder S, Nåsell H, et al. Effects of a perioperative smoking cessation intervention on postoperative complications: A randomized trial. Annals of Surgery. 2008;**248**(5):739-745

[58] Endara M, Masden D, Goldstein J, Gondek S, Steinberg J, Attinger C. The role of chronic and perioperative glucose management in high-risk surgical closures: A case for tighter glycemic control. Plastic and Reconstructive Surgery. 2013;**132**(4):996-1004

[59] Ramos M, Khalpey Z, Lipsitz S, Steinberg J, Panizales MT, Zinner M, et al. Relationship of perioperative hyperglycemia and postoperative infections in patients who undergo general and vascular surgery. Annals of Surgery. 2008;**248**(4):585-591

[60] Ata A, Lee J, Bestle SL, Desemone J, Stain SC. Postoperative hyperglycemia and surgical site infection in general surgery patients. Archives of Surgery. 2010;**145**(9):858-864

[61] Desai KA, Razavi SA, Hart AM, Thompson PW, Losken A. The effect of BMI on outcomes following complex abdominal wall reconstructions. Annals of Plastic Surgery. 2016;**76**(Suppl 4): S295-S297

[62] Giordano SA, Garvey PB, Baumann DP, Liu J, Butler CE. The impact of body mass index on abdominal wall reconstruction outcomes: A comparative study. Plastic and Reconstructive Surgery. 2017;**139**(5):1234-1244

Section 3

# Inguinal Hernia

Chapter 6

# The Tension-Free Repairs without Mesh: Desarda and Modified Bassini Techniques

*Frederica Jessie Tchoungui Ritz*

## Abstract

Hernia repair has three principal objectives: suppress the hernia, prevent recidivism, and reduce postoperative pain. Many techniques have been developed especially the tension-free repair. The Lichtenstein technique is the gold standard, using a mesh. However, sub-Saharan population is known to be hard laborers leading to the high-risk factor of acquiring hernia by a parietal defect. Most of them need a heterologous hernioplasty but have limited resources. The challenge in these countries is respecting the principal objectives of a hernia repair with inexpensive prosthetic material or without it. During these previous years, two principal techniques have been developed and used with satisfied results: Desarda and Modified Bassini techniques.

**Keywords:** inguinal hernia, Desarda, modified Bassini, Lichtenstein, tension-free repair

## 1. Introduction

Inguinal hernia is one of the common surgical pathologies. A better understanding of the anatomy of the inguinal canal improved the surgical techniques and the outcomes for the patients. Developed countries are well organized in scientific societies enhancing these improvements. Instead, the sub-Saharan countries do not have specialized centers which will help by improving the hernia surgery [1] and the general surgeon's training. The problematic of hernia surgery here is double, the improvement of inexpensive safe techniques and training of the general surgeons. This chapter emphasizes on two tension-free repair techniques, Desarda and modified Bassini, which are currently used for their low cost and are easily learned by the surgeons [2].

## 2. Modified Bassini repair

Bassini developed his hernia repair in 1887, which was minutely described by his student Catterina in 1930. This technique is the one currently used by general surgeon in secondary and tertiary hospitals in sub-Saharan countries. A modified Bassini was introduced, described as an autologous patch. The intervention can be under general or locoregional anesthesia. The description below is a modified Bassini technique by Atah [3].



IntechOpen

### 2.1 Technique

#### 2.1.1 Skin incision

A semi-Pfannenstiel incision is done homolateral to the hernia, for an esthetic scar. The inguinal canal opening is performed parallel to the inguinal ligament and the conjoint tendon through the superficial fascia and deep fascia; the external oblique aponeurosis (EOA) is cut. The EOA cut is extended to the superficial inguinal ring. The spermatic cord is opened layer by layer, and the hernia sac is exposed, dissected, and resected.

#### 2.1.2 Parietal repair

Through the inguinal canal, the internal oblique tendon and the transverse tendon are united to form the joint tendon or separated. Those muscle fibers are parallel to the external oblique muscle, which is behind them. The conjoint tendon or the internal oblique tendon is easily used to strengthen the inguinal canal.

The herniorrhaphy is made with the inguinal ligament left in its normal position without being dissected and sutured to the conjoint tendon with number 1 or 0 Polyglactin 910 rounded overlock suture. The suture begins at the pubic tubercle to the deep inguinal ring. The free leaf of the conjoint tendon is sutured to the inferior part of the inguinal ligament, behind the spermatic cordon following the retro-funicular Bassini technique.

The diameter of the deep inguinal ring is reduced with a separate point, to admit only the tip of the little finger, enough caring not to strangulate the spermatic cordon in male or the round ligament in female. If the repair is under tension, a discharge incision is done, and the two borders are sutured to the EOA with number 1 or 0 Polyglactin 910 interrupted sutures. The skin closure is done.

## 3. Desarda repair

The Desarda hernia repair, eponym name to its author, described in 2001, is an autologous hernioplasty. The technique was developed as a tension-free hernia repair without mesh, to reduce the chronic groin pain, recovery time, and cost [4]. The intervention can be performed under general anesthesia or locoregional anesthesia.

### 3.1 Technique

#### 3.1.1 Skin incision

The skin incision is a 6 cm oblique at the level of the inferior abdominal line or the Malgaigne's line (**Figure 1**). The fascia is incised and the EOA exposed. The EOA is cut in line with the inguinal ligament and the upper crux of the superficial ring, with a medial leaf and lateral leaf (**Figure 2**).

#### 3.1.2 Hernia sac dissection

A direct or indirect hernia, with or without a sac, can be found. The cremaster muscle is resected, and the hernia sac dissected in the direction of the deep inguinal ring protecting the spermatic cord (**Figure 3**). The sac is ligatured with a resorbable thread USP 2/0 and excised in an indirect hernia and inverted in a direct hernia.

*DOI: http://dx.doi.org/10.5772/intechopen.88955*

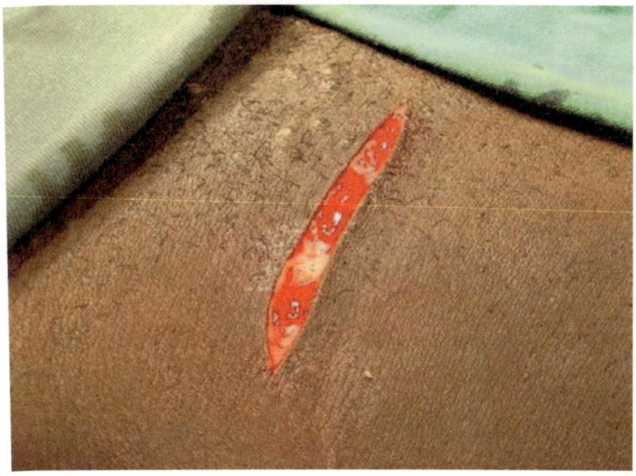

**Figure 1.**
*Skin incision.*

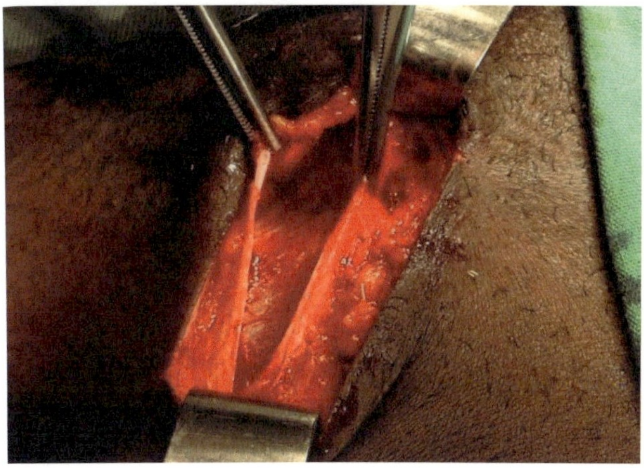

**Figure 2.**
*External oblique aponeurosis incision.*

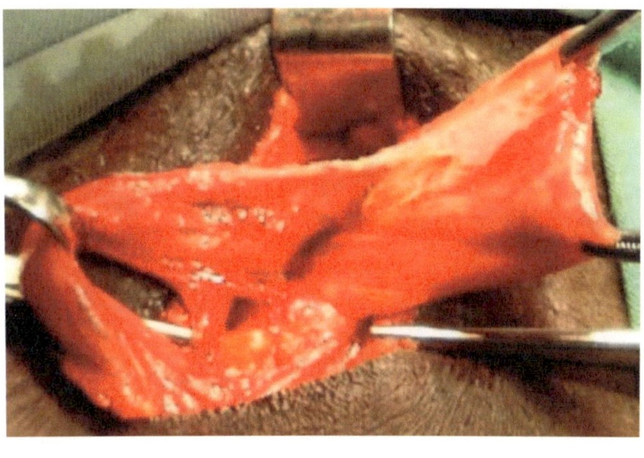

**Figure 3.**
*Hernia sac dissection.*

### 3.1.3 Parietal repair

The fascial plasty starts with the medial leaf of the EOA which is sutured with the inguinal ligament from the pubic tubercle to the abdominal ring using number 2/0 or 0 Monofilament Polydioxanone continuous sutures (**Figure 4**). The first two sutures were taken through the anterior rectus sheath, and the last suture is taken to narrow the abdominal ring sufficiently, caring not to strangulate the spermatic cord.

An incision is made on the sutured medial leaf to obtain an aponeurosis flap of 1–2 cm (**Figure 5**). This fascial flap is extended medially up to the pubic symphysis and 2 cm beyond the abdominal ring laterally.

The upper free border of the aponeurosis flap is sutured to the internal oblique muscle at the level of the conjoint tendon with a number 2/0 or 0 Monofilament Polydioxanone continuous suture (**Figure 6**). With these sutures of the EOA, a new posterior wall of the inguinal canal is formed behind the spermatic cord. After the suture of the EOA, the patient is asked to cough or strain if it is under locoregional anesthesia, and under general anesthesia the anesthetist is asked to give a deep breath to the patient; this is to verify the solidity of the new posterior wall.

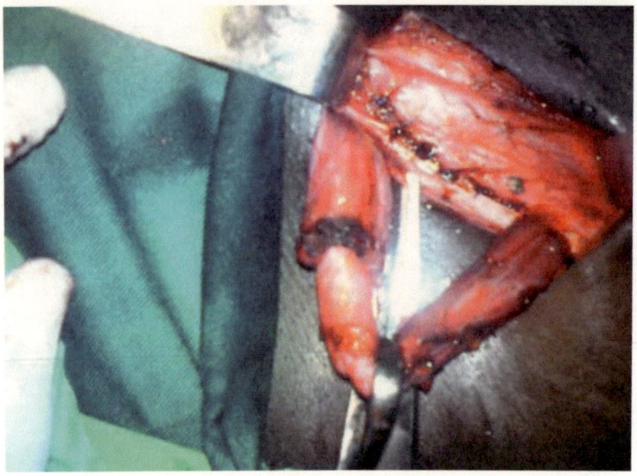

**Figure 4.**
*Suture of the medial leaf of the EOA to the inguinal ligament.*

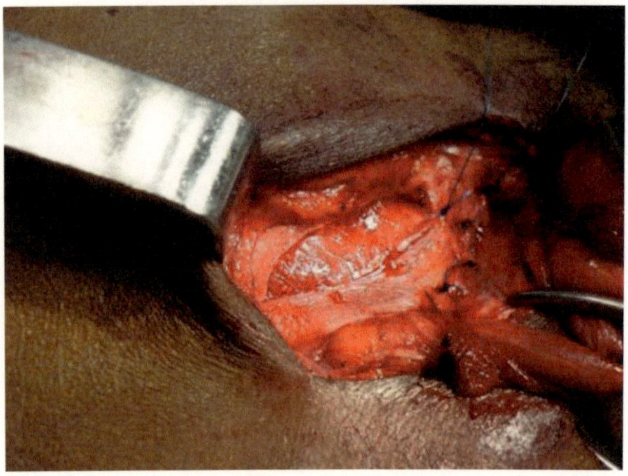

**Figure 5.**
*Incision of the sutured medial leaf of the EOA.*

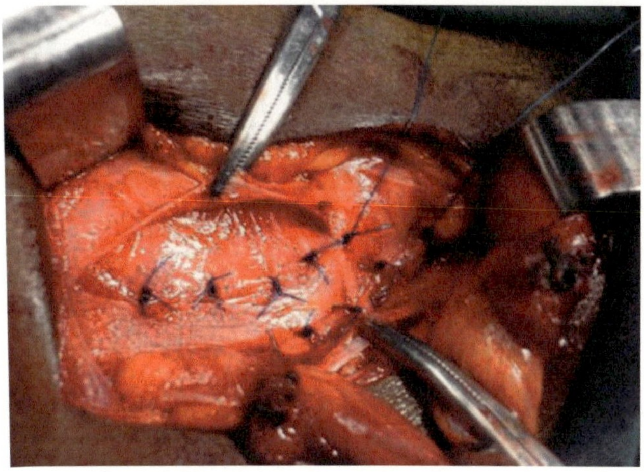

**Figure 6.**
*Suture of the upper free border of the aponeurosis flap.*

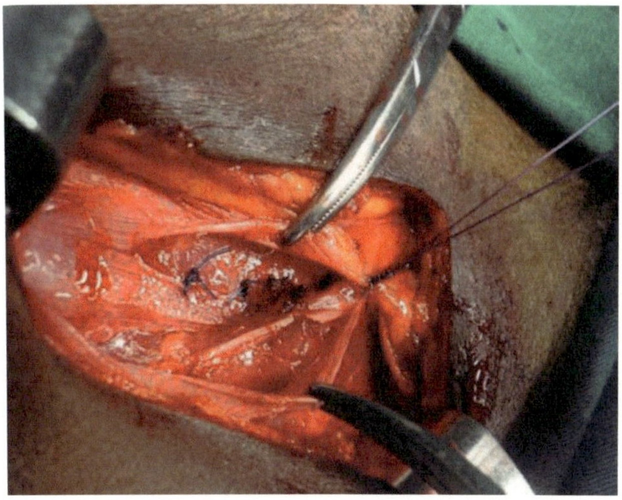

**Figure 7.**
*Suture of the lateral leaf of the EOA to the new medial leaf of the EOA.*

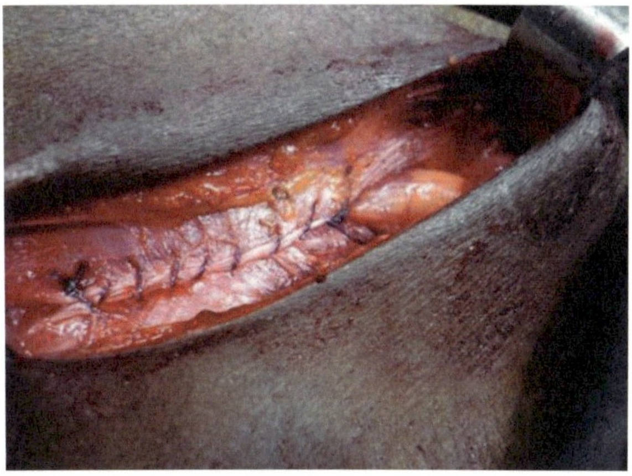

**Figure 8.**
*Closure of the EOA.*

The spermatic cord is replaced in the inguinal canal; the lateral leaf of the EOA is sutured to the new medial leaf of the EOA with a number 2/0 Monofilament Polydioxanone continuous sutures (**Figure 7**).

The EOA is sutured forward the spermatic cord (**Figure 8**), and a classic closure of the superficial fascia and the skin is done.

## 4. Results

The recurrence rate after an inguinal hernia repair is difficult to determine because of the high percentage of loss to follow-up. But some studies have shown that the modified Bassini technique is the most commonly used or the inguinal hernia repair [5]. This could be explained by the fact that surgeons in most of the peripheral hospitals are using tissue repair, mainly due to the limited resources of the population [6].

However, some complications occur with the tissue repair. Complications encountered in patient follow-up after a modified Bassini hernia repair are multiple; a prospective study in a rural hospital including 300 male patients highlighted some of them (**Table 1**).

The same complications can be observed with the Desarda technique as shown in a prospective study of 2 years, with 100 patients (**Table 2**) [7].

The two techniques are cost inexpensive, with a low rate of recurrence of the hernia and postoperative pain.

The European Hernia Society (EHS) gold standard regarding open tension-free hernia repair is the Lichtenstein mesh repair. However complications associated

| **Complications** | **Incidence (%)** |
|---|---|
| Urine retention | 5 (2.07) |
| Hematoma (superficial) | 1 (0.41) |
| Wound infection | 1 (0.41) |
| Seroma | 2 (0.83) |
| Postoperative neuralgia | 3 (1.24) |
| Scrotal edema | 2 (0.83) |
| Ischemic orchitis | 0 (0.00) |
| Recurrence | 2 (0.83) |

**Table 1.**
*Complications encountered with modified Bassini technique [6].*

| **Complications** | **Incidence (%)** |
|---|---|
| Urine retention | 3 (0.03) |
| Wound infection | 4 (0.04) |
| Vomiting | 2 (0.02) |
| Acute postoperative pain | 32 (0.32) |
| Chronic postoperative pain after 3 months | 4 (0.01) |
| Scrotal edema | 2 (0.02) |
| Recurrence from 3 to 27 months | 0 (0.00) |

**Table 2.**
*Complications encountered with Desarda technique.*

with it includes an important rate of mesh-related infection as wound infection due in some cases to an allergic reaction, mesh migration, and nerve entrapment [8]. These complications can lead to a prolonged hospital stay and a long treatment with antibiotics. Using Desarda or modified Bassini techniques avoid the risk of mesh-related complications, which would be an extra cost for the patient.

Inguinal hernia treatment depends also on the surgeon training and experiences. There are several tension-free techniques describe with or without mesh. Another goal in the management of hernias is the training of surgeons, depending on the medical and socioeconomic context.

## 5. Conclusion

Inguinal hernia is one of the commonest surgical pathology. In sub-Saharan Africa, it should be considered as a public health disease, to improve its management. The socioeconomic context is important here to consider the choice of the hernia repair technique. The tension-free repairs without mesh, Desarda and modified Bassini, response well to the economic criteria, with the advantages of a low rate of recurrence, postoperative pain, and reduced hospital stay.

## Conflict of interest

The author declared no potential conflicts of interest with respect to the research, authorship, and/or publication of this manuscript.

**Author details**

Frederica Jessie Tchoungui Ritz
Faculty of Medicine, Pharmacy and Odontology, Cheikh Anta Diop University, Dakar, Senegal

*Address all correspondence to: fredericatchoungui@gmail.com

## References

[1] Ohene-Yeboah M, Abantanga FA. Inguinal hernia disease in Africa: A common but neglected surgical condition. West African Journal of Medicine. 2011;**30**(2):77-83

[2] Kingsnorth AN, Clarke MG, Shillcutt SD. Public Health and Policy Issues of Hernia Surgery in Africa. World Journal of Surgery. 2009;**33**(6):1188. DOI: 10.1007/s00268-009-9964-y

[3] Mgba JA, Tangnyin CP, Atah TN, Meva'a JB, Sosso MA. Cure des Hernies Inguinales en Tension -Free (Nouvelle technique en Bassini modifiée). Health Sciences and Diseases. 2016;**17**(4):83-87

[4] Desarda MP. No-mesh inguinal hernia repair with continuous absorbable sutures: A dream or reality? (A study of 229 patients). Saudi Journal of Gastroenterology: Official Journal of the Saudi Gastroenterology Association. 2008;**14**(3):122-127

[5] Konate I. Primary unilateral uncomplicated inguinal hernia repair, which is the procedure most frequently, performed in operating theatres the world over? Situation of Africa. Hernia. Jun 2019;**23**(3):623-624. DOI: 10.1007/s10029-019-01937-5. [Epub 9 May 2019]

[6] Gorad K, Lohar H, Patil S, Tonape T, Gautam R. Modified Bassini's repair: Our experience in a rural hospital setup. Medical Journal of Dr. DY Patil University. 2013;**6**:378. DOI: 10.4103/0975-2870.118276

[7] Dieng M, Cissé M, Seck M, Diallo F, Touré A, Konaté I, et al. Cure des hernies inguinales simples de l'adulte par plastie avec l'aponévrose du grand oblique: Technique de Desarda. e-mémoires de l'Académie Nationale de Chirurgie. 2012;**11**(2):069-074

[8] Zulu HG, Mewa Kinoo S, Singh B. Comparison of Lichtenstein inguinal hernia repair with the tension-free Desarda technique: a clinical audit and review of the literature. Tropical Doctor. 2016;**46**(3):125-129

Chapter 7

# Mesh Fixation Methods in Groin Hernia Surgery

*Morena Burati, Alberto Scaini, Luca Andrea Fumagalli, Francesco Gabrielli and Marco Chiarelli*

## Abstract

No unanimous consent has been reached by surgeons in terms of a method for mesh fixation in laparoscopic and open surgery for inguinal hernia repair. Many different methods of fixation are available, and the choice of which one to use is still based on surgeons' preferences. At present, tissue glues, sutures, and laparoscopic tacks are the most common fixating methods. In open technique, sutures have been the method of choice for their reduced costs and surgeons' habits. Nevertheless, tissue glues have been demonstrated to be effective and safe. Similarly, tacks can be considered the most common means of fixation in laparoscopic hernia repair, but they are connected to a higher risk of complication and morbidity. In this chapter, we present these types of mesh fixation, their characteristics and potential risks, and advantages of their use.

**Keywords:** inguinal hernia, mesh, fixation, fixation techniques, fibrin glue, cyanoacrylic glue, tacks, suture

## 1. Introduction

Inguinal hernia repair is one of the most common procedures in surgical practice. In the surgical repair of groin hernia, prosthetic meshes and their fixation have been subject to debate. In the last decades, synthetic meshes have become crucial in surgical treatment of inguinal hernia. Once positioned, meshes are designed to be integrated in local tissue by a fibrotic reaction that gradually incorporates them. Therefore, a good fixation is essential to secure the mesh in its correct position, while the integration process occurs.

The introduction of synthetic meshes and their proper fixation has reduced recurrence rates to below 5%. As a consequence, the most frequent postoperative morbidities have become mesh migration, chronic pain, infection, and seroma [1, 2]. In surgical practice the main challenge in mesh fixation consists in finding a good balance between the strength of fixation, in order to avoid recurrence and the risk of tissue trauma and nerve entrapment, leading to chronic pain.

At present, various fixation techniques and materials have been developed, but no unanimous consent has been reached on the "best" method of fixation. The choice is still based on surgeon's preferences and experience, and much still depends on local habits and personal beliefs.

## 2. Mesh fixation

### 2.1 Fixation methods

The primary function of a fixation device is to keep the mesh in place until tissue ingrowth is completed. The interaction between mesh and tissue depends on the type of mesh; however, complete integration is usually achieved within 2–3 weeks after surgery. It is important to underline that shear strength is reached for 74% during the first 2 weeks. Until then, therefore, proper fixation is essential. Different types of fixation medium can be used in inguinal hernia surgery, the main ones being tissue glues, staples and tacks, and sutures.

#### *2.1.1 Tissue glues*

Tissue adhesives have been introduced in medical practice during the 1960s. Since then, they have been used in numerous procedures like skin closure, suture reinforcement, arteriovenous embolization, endoscopic treatment of ulcers and varices, and fixation of meshes in abdominal wall defect repair.

Two types of tissue adhesive for mesh fixation are available in surgical practice:

##### *2.1.1.1 Fibrin glues (Tisseel®, Tissucol®, and Evicel®)*

It is made of four components: human purified fibrinogen, bovine atropine solution, human thrombin, and calcium chloride. Alongside its hemostatic action, the fibrinogen component gives the product tensile strength and adhesive properties. It also promotes fibroblast proliferation [3]. These are mixed at the time of fixation to duplicate the terminal coagulation reaction and generate polymerized fibrin [4]. Once applied to the mesh, 3 min may be required to complete the reaction [5].

##### *2.1.1.2 Cyanoacrylic tissue glues (Histoacryl®, Glubran®, and Glubran-2®)*

These glues are synthetic (n-butyl-cyanoacrylate) or hybrid tissue sealants. They are known for strong and rapid adhesive properties. Cyanoacrylic glues ensure high-degree and strong bonding to biologic tissues when compared with other adhesives. When they get in contact with blood or water contained in the tissue, they form a very tight cover, binding to the surface within 5–6 s [6]. Glubran-2 is the most recently produced tissue adhesive. Its peculiarity is a longer radical chain with a lower temperature of polymerization compared to Histoacryl®, which results in lower toxicity and fewer inflammatory reactions [7].

At present, there is no evidence in medical literature as to which glue may be considered better in mesh fixation during inguinal hernia repair. Nevertheless, it must be remarked that using glue for mesh fixation increases the costs of hernioplasty, if compared with sutures.

#### *2.1.2 Tacks*

Tack fixation has been performed since the introduction of laparoscopic inguinal and ventral hernia repair between the late 1980s and the early 1990s. In current practice, three types of tacks are commonly used, divided into two categories: absorbable and nonabsorbable.

#### 2.1.2.1 Helical titanium tacks (ProTack®)

It is a laparoscopic device, which places a helical coil into the fascia and muscle of the anterior abdominal wall. The tack itself has a helical shape, measures 4 mm in length and 3 mm in width, and penetrates approximately 3–4 mm into these tissues. To be placed correctly, tacks must be placed 1–1.5 cm apart, along the periphery of the mesh [8].

#### 2.1.2.2 Helical nontitanium tacks (PermaFix®)

These tacks are made of polyacetal, a molded, polymer-based material. It is a permanent hollow tack with an atraumatic tip, 6.7 mm long [9].

#### 2.1.2.3 Absorbable tacks (AbsorbaTack®, PermaSorb®, and SorbaFix®)

These tacks are made of polymers or copolymers (poly(D,L)-lactide or glycolide-co-L-lactide). They measure between 6.4 and 6.7 mm and adsorb in 12–16 months [9].

Overall, tacks provide an excellent fixation strength, and they are also easy to apply. Nevertheless, their use is associated with significant morbidity. The penetration of the abdominal wall, in fact, may cause nerve and vessel entrapment. Also, tacks are themselves foreign bodies introduced in the abdomen, so they may cause inflammatory reactions. As a result, a significant number of patients suffer from pain and develop adhesion in the postoperative period. Moreover, cases of migration of titanium tacks have been described. At present, absorbable tacks are connected to lower inflammation rates, adhesion formation, and migration so the use of titanium tacks is no longer advisable.

### 2.1.3 Sutures

Sutures commonly used in hernia repair are divided into two: absorbable and nonabsorbable, each characterized by a different degree of tension generated and a different time of strength loss due to degradation.

#### 2.1.3.1 Absorbable sutures (poliglecaprone (Monocryl®), polyglactin (Vicryl®), polyglycolic acid (Dexon®), polyglyconate (Maxon®), and polydioxanone (PDS®))

Their loss of strength has been classified and varies from a minimum of 1 week (Monocryl®) to a maximum of 4–5 weeks (PDS®).

#### 2.1.3.2 Nonabsorbable sutures (polypropylene (Prolene®) and polyamide (Nylon))

These sutures are designed to retain most of their strength indefinitely.

International medical literature offers evidence that both absorbable and nonabsorbable sutures seem to provide enough strength and tension to prevent recurrence. International randomized trials do not seem to highlight significant difference between the two types of sutures in terms of postoperative complications.

Nevertheless, nonabsorbable suture seems to be connected to a higher incidence of postoperative pain due to entrapment of a nerve by suture or mesh [10].

## 2.2 Mesh fixation and surgical techniques

As mentioned above, several mesh fixation methods exist, including tacks, staples, self-fixing, fibrin sealants, synthetic glues, and sutures. Which method to choose to secure a mesh during surgical hernia repair depends on many factors such as personal beliefs, local habits and "dogmas," type of the hernia, and size of the defect but, most of all, on surgical technique.

Two approaches to repair inguinal hernia are common practice in surgery: the open approach, usually the Lichtenstein technique, and the laparoscopic approach, meaning both preperitoneal and extraperitoneal repair.

### *2.2.1 Open technique*

Groin hernioplasty is the most common operation in general surgery. Due to its lower costs, shorter operating times, and reduced complication risks, the open Lichtenstein technique is performed more frequently. Lichtenstein hernia repair, in fact, is simple, safe, and easy to learn, with very good results in terms of morbidity and a very low recurrence rate.

Both sutures (absorbable and nonabsorbable) and glues (fibrin and cyanoacrylic) can be used to seal the mesh to the abdominal wall.

According to standard operating technique, once the mesh is placed and adjusted, the upper edge is kept in place with two or three sutures, one to the rectus sheath and the others to the internal oblique aponeurosis. Also the lower lateral edges of each of the two tails of the mesh are fixed to the inguinal ligament, leaving enough space for the passage of the spermatic cord.

The use of tissue adhesive to secure the mesh has become an internationally accepted practice in the last few decades. In the sutureless technique, the mesh is fixated by using fibrin or cyanoacrylic glue, whose components get mixed during the operation. Once activated, the glue is poured beneath the mesh, covering the whole Hesselbach's triangle. The mesh is placed above the glue and pressed against the inguinal floor for about 2 min [11].

Suture mesh fixation in inguinal hernia repair represents the main source of complications, possibly leading to inflammation and surgical site infection (SSI), hematoma, nerve entrapment, and chronic pain.

A 2014 systematic review including 12 articles by Sanders et al. [12] found an infection rate between 0 and 3.5%, and no significant difference in terms of SSIs incidence was detected between the groups. Anyway, there is no study specifying the depth of infection, whether it was deep or superficial. This could lead to improper conclusions, being a deep infection more related to the presence of the mesh.

Pain is a very important outcome after surgical repair of groin hernia. Pain is defined as acute, when it occurs in the first week after the operation, and chronic, when it lasts beyond 3 months after surgery. Two RCTs, recently published in medical literature, have demonstrated a significant lower incidence of acute pain after using fibrin sealant ($p < 0.001$) [13] and cyanoacrylic glue ($p < 0.003$) [14] compared to suture fixation.

A recent meta-analyses, including 13 RCTs comparing glue versus suture mesh fixation in Lichtenstein inguinal hernia repair [15, 16], showed a lower incidence of early acute pain ($p = 0.03$) and hematoma in the glue fixation group. On the other hand, chronic pain is one of the main issues after hernioplasty, and sutureless techniques were introduced in surgery in an attempt to reduce its incidence, without affecting recurrence rates. According to the international guidelines for groin hernia management, the incidence of chronic pain ranges from 0 to 36.3% [17]. In particular, 14.7% is for sutures, 7.6% for cyanoacrylic glues, and 3.7% for fibrin glues. Three international RCTs suggest that the use of fibrin or cyanoacrylic glue can reduce pain if compared to suture [10, 12]. In particular, the TIMELI international trial demonstrated that fibrin glue was connected to the reduction of chronic symptoms like numbness and discomfort after 1 year.

Among the possible complications, recurrence is possibly the one that concerns surgeons the most. According to Sanders et al.'s review, recurrence rate is 1.3%. There was no significant difference between fixation methods in any of the RCTs, although long-term recurrence rates have not been determined and large hernias often have been excluded.

Concluding, in open inguinal hernia repair, no differences in recurrence or surgical site infection between different mesh fixation methods have been reported in literature, while sutureless fixation may reduce the onset of acute and chronic pain. Therefore, according to HerniaSurge Group consensus, glue fixation in the Lichtenstein technique can be performed in direct or indirect hernias less than 3 cm large (MII or LII types, EHS classification).

### 2.2.2 *Laparoscopic technique*

At present, the two most common laparoscopic techniques for hernia repair are the transabdominal preperitoneal repair (TAPP) and the total extraperitoneal repair (TEP). Both techniques involve the placement of a mesh in the preperitoneal space that must cover all potential hernia sites. The mesh in the preperitoneal space is subject to intra-abdominal forces and may be easily displaced before fibrosis seals it to the inguinal canal. In particular, the medial edge of the mesh is most susceptible to displacement, leading to inevitable recurrence if the medial part of the inguinal canal gets exposed. This underlines the importance of fixation [18]. Tacks, glues, and sutures can all be used to fixate the mesh.

Arguably, the most popular technique among surgeons is the use of tacks. However, it is known that using tacks and staples to secure the mesh can lead to complications, such as chronic pain. During the mesh fixation, in fact, it is really important not to place any tack or staple below the iliopubic tract, avoiding the triangle of pain. Lateral fixation should also be avoided, to prevent inadvertent damage to the nerves. Also misplaced tacks are described in literature to be responsible for nerve irritation and injury. The alternatives of the use of tacks are tissue glues and sutures.

Sutures usually require expertise and longer operating times. Both absorbable and nonabsorbable sutures may be used to fixate mesh to the abdominal wall. Sutures are usually applied transfascially after reduction of intraperitoneal pressure. Suture type, quantity, and placement vary among surgeons and no "gold standard" technique has been established [19].

Tissue glues have been introduced in laparoscopic hernia repair to reduce morbidity, such as pain and hematoma, thanks to their atraumatic application and their hemostatic properties [20].

Several studies, including meta-analyses and RCTs, comparing complication rates after different fixation methods, have been produced.

Complications after TEP repair, using tacks against glue, have been analyzed in a recent review by Kaul et al. [21]. The authors included in the study four RCTs for a total of 664 procedures. According to their results, no significant difference in terms of SSIs rates could be registered.

Acute pain after TEP was analyzed in a randomized prospective trial by Lau in [22]. The study concluded that, even if glue group consumed significantly less analgesics compared to staple group (p = 0.034), no significant difference has been registered in the postoperative pain score in the first week after surgery. On the other hand, Kaul et al.'s review reported a significant difference in terms of chronic pain incidence between the two groups (OR 3.25; 95% CI 1.62–6.49).

As already said, recurrence is a very important outcome when it comes to inguinal hernia repair. According to the two meta-analyses present in literature, there is no evidence of a significant difference in terms of recurrence, after using tissue sealants or tacks to fix the mesh [21, 23].

Similar results can be found in literature about TAPP technique. In a recent meta-analyses by Shah et al. [24], including five randomized controlled trials and five non-RCTs, no significant differences were found in terms of acute pain, SSIs, or recurrence. Nevertheless, patients who underwent TAPP hernia repair, using tissue sealant for mesh fixation, experienced significant less chronic pain (p = 0.005). Several RCTs published in the last decade have confirmed these findings [25–27].

Concluding, international RCTs and several meta-analyses have proven tissue glue to be as safe as tacks in terms of recurrence and SSI. In addition, chronic pain was significantly less represented when tissue adhesives were used for the fixation of the mesh. Therefore, according to international guidelines, to minimize the risk of acute postoperative pain, atraumatic fixation techniques (fibrin glue, cyanoacrylate) should be considered.

## 3. Conclusions

When it comes to mesh fixation, no unanimous consent about technique has ever been reached. Several types of fixation methods exist such as tacks, staples, self-fixing, fibrin sealants, glues, and sutures. The choice of which method to use strongly depends on the type of surgery and the type of defect but also (and often decisively) on surgeons' personal beliefs and local habits. In open technique both sutures and tissue adhesives have been proven equally safe in terms of recurrence and wound infection, but glues are connected to less chronic pain onset. Therefore, glue fixation in the Lichtenstein technique can be performed in MII or LII types (EHS classification) hernias.

Similarly, in the laparoscopic approach, tacks or glues can be used to secure the mesh showing similar recurrence rates. Again, adhesive fixation is connected to less morbidity in terms of chronic pain.

In conclusion, international RCTs and recent meta-analyses have confirmed tissue adhesives to be a valid alternative to traditional sutures and tacks. When it comes to the choice of which fixation procedure to perform in inguinal hernia repair, many authors advise the use of tissue sealants to minimize the risks of chronic pain, justifying the higher costs due to the use of expensive glues.

## Acknowledgements

Morena Burati MD: project conception; acquisition; analysis; and interpretation of data and drafting of the work. Marco Chiarelli MD: project design; acquisition; interpretation of data; and revising of the work.

Alberto Scaini MD: project design; acquisition; and interpretation of data.

Luca Andrea Fumagalli MD: project design; acquisition; and interpretation of data.

Francesco Gabrielli PhD: project design; acquisition; interpretation of data; and revising of the work.

## Conflict of interest

The authors do not have any conflict of interest.

## Author details

Morena Burati[1]*, Alberto Scaini[1], Luca Andrea Fumagalli[1], Francesco Gabrielli[2,3] and Marco Chiarelli[1]

1 Emergency and Robotic Surgery Department, A. Manzoni Hospital, Lecco, LC, Italy

2 University Milano-Bicocca, Milan, Italy

3 General Surgery Department, Istituti Clinici Zucchi, Monza, MB, Italy

*Address all correspondence to: morena.burati@gmail.com

## References

[1] Hoyuela C et al. Randomized clinical trial of mesh fixation with glue or sutures for Lichtenstein hernia repair. The British Journal of Surgery. 2017;**104**(6):688-694

[2] Guttadauro A et al. 'All-in-one mesh' hernioplasty: A new procedure for primary inguinal hernia open repair. Asian Journal of Surgery. 2018;**41**(5):473-479

[3] Katkhouda N et al. Use of fibrin sealant for prosthetic mesh fixation in laparoscopic extraperitoneal inguinal hernia repair. Annals of Surgery. 2001;**233**(1):18-25

[4] Olmi S, Scaini A, Erba L, Bertolini A, Croce E. Laparoscopic repair of inguinal hernias using an intraperitoneal onlay mesh technique and a Parietex composite mesh fixed with fibrin glue (Tissucol). Personal technique and preliminary results. Surgical Endoscopy. 2007;**21**(11):1961-1964

[5] Campanelli G et al. Randomized, controlled, blinded trial of Tisseel/Tissucol for mesh fixation in patients undergoing Lichtenstein technique for primary inguinal hernia repair: Results of the TIMELI trial. Annals of Surgery. 2012;**255**(4):650-657

[6] Ayyıldız SN, Ayyıldız A. Cyanoacrylic tissue glues: Biochemical properties and their usage in urology. Turkish Journal of Urology. 2017;**43**(1):14-24

[7] Montanaro L et al. Cytotoxicity, blood compatibility and antimicrobial activity of two cyanoacrylate glues for surgical use. Biomaterials. 2000;**22**(1):59-66

[8] LeBlanc KA. Tack hernia: A new entity. JSLS - Journal of the Society of Laparoendscopic Surgeons. 2003;7(4):383-387

[9] Reynvoet E, Berrevoet F. Pros and cons of tacking in laparoscopic hernia repair. Surgical Technology International. 2014;**25**:136-140

[10] Dobrin PB. Suture selection for hernia repair. In: Abdominal Wall Hernias. New York, NY: Springer New York; 2001. pp. 237-245

[11] Sun P, Cheng X, Hu Q, Zheng Q, Deng S, Sun Y. Mesh fixation with glue versus suture for chronic pain and recurrence in Lichtenstein inguinal hernioplasty. Cochrane Database of Systematic Reviews. 2017;**2**:2017

[12] Sanders DL, Waydia S. A systematic review of randomised control trials assessing mesh fixation in open inguinal hernia repair. Hernia. 2014;**18**(2):165-176

[13] Lionetti R, Neola B, Dilillo S, Bruzzese D, Ferulano GP. Sutureless hernioplasty with light-weight mesh and fibrin glue versus Lichtenstein procedure: A comparison of outcomes focusing on chronic postoperative pain. Hernia. 2012;**16**(2):127-131

[14] Nowobilski W, Dobosz M, Wojciechowicz T, Mionskowska L. Lichtenstein inguinal hernioplasty using butyl-2-cyanoacrylate versus sutures. Preliminary experience of a prospective randomized trial. European Surgical Research. 2004;**36**(6):367-370

[15] Lin H, Zhuang Z, Ma T, Sun X, Huang X, Li Y. A meta-analysis of randomized control trials assessing mesh fixation with glue versus suture in Lichtenstein inguinal hernia repair. Medicine (Baltimore). 2018;**97**(14):1-9

[16] Shen Y, Sun W, Chen J, Liu S, Wang M. NBCA medical adhesive (n-butyl-2-cyanoacrylate) versus suture for patch fixation in Lichtenstein inguinal herniorrhaphy: A

randomized controlled trial. Surgery. 2012;**151**(4):550-555

[17] Simons MP et al. International guidelines for groin hernia management. Hernia. 2018;**22**(1):1-165

[18] Jacob BP, Ramshaw B. The SAGES Manual of Hernia Repair. Springer; 2013

[19] Sucher JF, Klebuc M. Abdominal wall hernias. Common Problems in Acute Care Surgery. 2013;**55**(2018):421-440

[20] Olmi S, Erba L, Bertolini A, Scaini A, Croce E. Fibrin glue for mesh fixation in laparoscopic transabdominal preperitoneal (TAPP) hernia repair: Indications, technique, and outcomes. Surgical Endoscopy. 2006;**20**(12):1846-1850

[21] Kaul A et al. Staple versus fibrin glue fixation in laparoscopic total extraperitoneal repair of inguinal hernia: A systematic review and meta-analysis. Surgical Endoscopy. 2012;**26**(5):1269-1278

[22] Lau H. Fibrin sealant versus mechanical stapling for mesh fixation during endoscopic extraperitoneal inguinal hernioplasty. Annals of Surgery. 2005;**242**(5):670-675

[23] Sajid MS, Ladwa N, Kalra L, McFall M, Baig MK, Sains P. A meta-analysis examining the use of tacker mesh fixation versus glue mesh fixation in laparoscopic inguinal hernia repair. American Journal of Surgery. 2013;**206**(1):103-111

[24] Shah NS, Fullwood C, Siriwardena AK, Sheen AJ. Mesh fixation at laparoscopic inguinal hernia repair: A meta-analysis comparing tissue glue and tack fixation. World Journal of Surgery. 2015;**38**(10):2558-2570

[25] Brügger L, Bloesch M, Ipaktchi R, Kurmann A, Candinas D, Beldi G. Objective hypoesthesia and pain after transabdominal preperitoneal hernioplasty: A prospective, randomized study comparing tissue adhesive versus spiral tacks. Surgical Endoscopy. 2012;**26**(4):1079-1085

[26] Tolver MA, Rosenberg J, Juul P, Bisgaard T. Randomized clinical trial of fibrin glue versus tacked fixation in laparoscopic groin hernia repair. Surgical Endoscopy. 2013;**27**(8):2727-2733

[27] Chan MS et al. Randomized double-blinded prospective trial of fibrin sealant spray versus mechanical stapling in laparoscopic total extraperitoneal hernioplasty. Annals of Surgery. 2014;**259**(3):432-437

Chapter 8

# New Laparoscopic Surgery in Inguinal Hernia Repair

*Reno Rudiman and Andika August Winata*


## Abstract

Laparoscopic inguinal herniorrhaphy has become widely accepted as an effective alternative to the treatment of hernias with the anterior approach. It has success rates identical to those of the conventional method and quickens recovery by decreasing time until return to work or physical activities. With the introduction of single incision laparoscopic surgery (SILS), there has been an exponential increase in the number of SILS hernia repair. It probably represents the single most exciting innovation in laparoscopic surgery of the last 2 decades. The main premise of SILS is the use of completely blunt ports, which will negate the risks of bowel and vascular injuries, less wound, less postoperative pain, cosmetically more favorable and lower the recurrent rate.


**Keywords:** inguinal hernia, laparoscopic, TAPP, TEP, SILS

## 1. Introduction

Surgery to treat various diseases has been recorded back to middle ages. For two centuries, large incisions were necessary to perform abdominal surgical procedures. Although effective, several known morbidities were related to this method, including postoperative pain, wound infection, incisional hernia, and prolonged hospitalization [1]. The present surgical site infection rate is 15–25%, depending on the level of contamination [2].

Laparoscopic surgery was introduced in 1983 by Lukichev and 1985 by Muhe who performed laparoscopic cholecystectomy. Their cumbersome techniques did not receive the attention they probably deserved. Interests were started to grow after Mouret in 1987 reported the first acknowledged laparoscopic cholecystectomy by means of four trocars [3]. Since then, operative laparoscopy has advanced progressively. Several operative procedures have been performed by this new approach. Due to its minimal invasiveness to abdominal wall, laparoscopic surgery is also called minimally invasive surgery. Laparoscopic procedures can be performed using small incisions of around 0.5–1.5 cm that can be made far away from the surgical site [4].

One of the main advantages of laparoscopic surgery over traditional open surgery is it often requires a shorter hospital stay than traditional open surgery. Procedure such as appendectomy or cholecystectomy is commonly stay at the hospital for only one night after surgery. This is due to patients are experiencing less pain and bleeding after surgery [5].

Another important advantage of laparoscopic surgery is that as the incision wound is so much smaller than open surgery, post-surgical scarring is significantly reduced. Cosmetically, it is more desirable to most patients. Risks of keloid forming are therefore significantly reduced as well [6].

In conventional laparoscopic surgery, three to four small incisions are made. In a more complex procedure such as large bowel resection or bariatric (obesity) surgery, up to six incisions can be made, allowing more instruments to be used to assist organ resection [4, 7–9]. Obviously, the more wounds are made, the more pain it will eventually be caused to the patients. On the contrary, less wound signifies less pain. This brings about the concept of single incision laparoscopic surgery [10, 11].

## 2. Laparoscopic hernia repair

Transabdominal preperitoneal (TAPP) repair and totally extraperitoneal (TEP) repair are the most common laparoscopic inguinal hernia repair techniques, since the early of 1990s [6]. In TAPP, the peritoneal cavity is explored by the surgeon and then a mesh is placed through a peritoneal incision over possible hernia sites. TEP is different as the peritoneal cavity is not penetrated and mesh is employed to seal the hernia from outside of the peritoneum [8]. Both techniques try to diminish the hernia and hernia sac within the abdomen and then place a 10 × 15 cm mesh just deep to the abdominal wall [12].

The more superior surgical approach and technique for inguinal hernia repair is still widely argued. TAPP laparoscopic inguinal hernia repair improved clinical outcome and associated with a better quality of patient's life in numerous study [13]. The advantages of this approach are capability to inspect abdominal cavity, excellent exposure and enabling bilateral repair if necessary. The disadvantages are the possibility of intraperitoneal structures injury, adhesion formation and possibility of late bowel obstruction [14] (**Figures 1** and **2**).

Peritoneal integrity preservation is the main reason for TEP laparoscopic inguinal hernia repair is preferred to the TAPP repair. However, the peculiarity of anatomy and working area restriction in general made it to be more difficult [15]. In TEP, the surgeon is able to create a space just deep to the abdominal muscles without entering the peritoneal cavity and minimizing adhesion formation [14, 16].

It has been more than 20 years since TAPP and TEP were introduced to clinical routine [17]. TEP is considered to be more difficult than TAPP but may have fewer complications [8].

Rhambia et al. in 2016 also conducted a comparative study between these techniques; they found that there is no significant difference between them in the

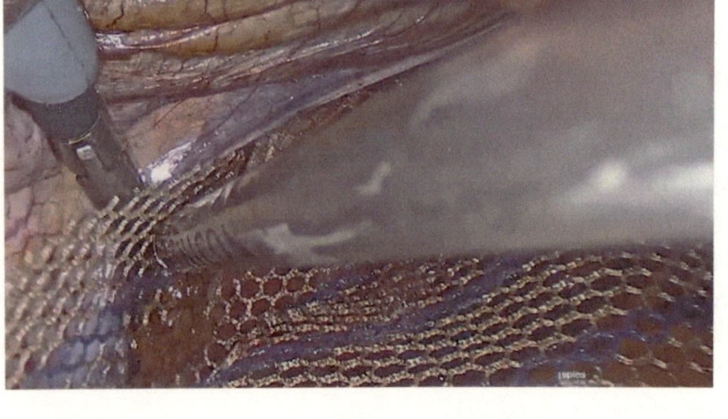

**Figure 1.**
*Positioning the mesh in inguinal area.*

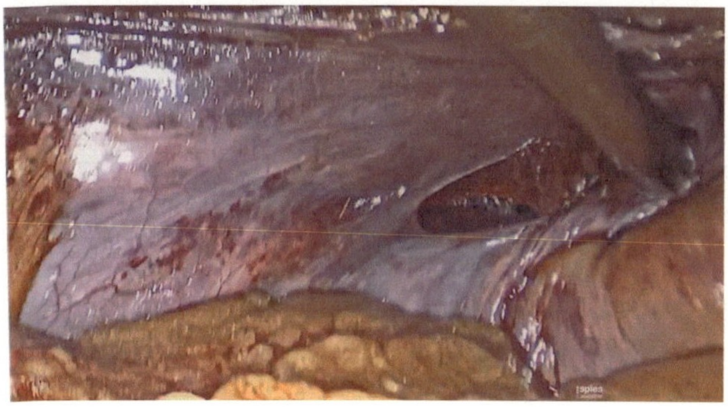

**Figure 2.**
*Peritoneum is closed.*

variable of duration of surgery, serious adverse event, persisting post-operative pain, hematoma, seroma, persisting numbness, hernia recurrence, port site of hernia and length of hospital stay. TEP gave the patients less pain after 24 hours of surgery in this research [18].

Former research by McCormack revealed that TAPP has slightly increased the number of hernias developing close by and injuries to internal organs. TEP has been associated with more conversions to another type of surgery. These are widely consistent results. Comparing these two techniques, the number of vascular injuries and deep and mesh infections is infrequent and there were no overt difference [8].

Apart from that, assuming a comparable patient group, identical indication and adequately experienced surgeons, similar results can be achieved with the TEP and TAPP technique. That is borne out by the comparable reoperation rate for postoperative complications [17].

### 2.1 SILS in hernia repair

An effective alternative to treat hernias is SILS that was introduced in 2007 after a port by Covidien was released. It is now probably represents the single most exciting innovation in laparoscopic surgery of the last 2 decades [19]. In hernia repair, SILS also accommodates TAPP or TEP to repair the defect. Early outcomes of this novel technique show it to be feasible, safe and with potentially better cosmetic outcome [20].

With this technique, the surgeon operates exclusively through a single entry point, typically at the patient's umbilicus. Unlike a traditional multi-port laparoscopic approach, SILS leaves only a single small scar [10, 21, 22]. During the introduction years on SILS in 1997, enthusiasm was limited because of lack of technical support and poor equipment [3]. In 2005, Hirano et al. reintroduced the technique with some advancements compared to previous technique. Since then, the technology was progressing steadily. Among advancements created were articulating instruments, laparoscope adjustments, several trocars adjacent into each other through a single incision [23].

SILS is gaining popularity due to its advantages in minimizing the invasiveness of surgical incisions. With the reduced number of incisions, the associated possible wound morbidities will also be reduced. This includes the reduced risks of wound infection, pain, bleeding, organ injury, and port site hernia [24]. In addition, one important feature of SILS is since the wound is at umbilicus, it leaves a single small scar that is well-hidden, it is almost unseen when the wound is healed, thereby it is almost "scarless" [10, 21, 25, 26].

In general, SILS techniques take about the same amount of time to do as traditional laparoscopic surgeries. However, SILS is recognized as to be a more complicated procedure because it involves manipulating three articulating instruments through one access port [22, 27, 28]. SILS performed with a similar technique to the conventional laparoscopic through a single umbilical port. The SILS-Port was introduced through a single 2.0–3.0 cm transverse transumbilical skin and facial incision. After creation of pneumoperitoneum at pressure of 12 mmHg, two 5-mm working ports and a 10-mm camera port was inserted. The peritoneal flap was prepared. A mesh was placed, and the peritoneum was closed with standard laparoscopic instruments or tackers. After releasing the pneumoperitoneum, the umbilical fascia was routinely closed with polypropylene loop suture and the skin was sutured with 4-0 absorbable intradermic sutures [29].

From financial point of view, the use of a single-port device and the increased skills needed to perform, SILS is slightly more costly to conventional multi-port laparoscopic surgery [25–27]. Generally, the length of stay in the hospital is shorter and the need of medical assistance is lesser than traditional laparoscopic surgeries [30].

Although SILS offers benefits for patients undergoing abdominal surgery, not everyone is an applicant for the procedure. Obesity, severe adhesions, or scarring from previous surgeries are a few of the factors that would prohibit patients from getting the surgery [26]. Nonetheless, new technologies are evolving continuously [27].

### *2.1.1 SILS versus conventional laparoscopic hernia repair*

A concordant evolution and improvement of the laparoscopic method has occurred when the advantages of minimally invasive surgical techniques are continuing to be defined. The less scar initiative has driven to a reduction in the number of port sites. Consequently, SILS is more popular and widely being used. As the findings show, repair of abdominal wall defects, specifically inguinal hernias, is feasible via SILS as well [31].

There are many studies comparing these two methods now. In Rajapandian et al. study, they assess the potential benefits of SILS without using specialized ports or instruments and compare the same with the conventional laparoscopic surgery in terms of operative time, post-operative pain, complications, cost and scars. They found that the mean duration of surgery was significantly longer in SILS for unilateral as well as bilateral hernia repair than its conventional counterpart. While the mean blood loss was comparable in either groups, various complications like vascular injury, peritoneal tear, cord and nerve injuries had not significant differences. In SILS, two patients were converted to conventional laparoscopy, but without any open conversion [26].

Ece et al. did a research from 148 patients, 88 underwent conventional laparoscopic repair and 60 underwent SILS repair. All SILS procedures were completed successfully without conversion conventional laparoscopic or open repair, and no additional port was required in both groups. There were no differences in operative time, length of hospital stay and VAS scores of patients 24 hours after the operation. No intraoperative major complications were observed such as vessel, intestine, or bladder injury. One patient in each group had a complaint of pain for longer than 3 months. Short-term complication rates were similar in each group. Several small seroma and hematomas were reported in both groups, and all of them were resolved with conservative treatment. Also, three patients treated with oral antibiotics for port site infection. Long-term complications such as mesh infection and recurrence were not detected in both the groups. Three patients in the SILS-TAPP group experienced port site hernia. All of the port site hernias were confirmed by ultrasound, and elective mesh hernioplasty was performed [29].

Another research by Buckley in 2014 described a slightly different result. SILS for unilateral cases was significantly shorter statistically than for conventional one. For bilateral cases, the average operative times for both were similar. No conversions from SILS to conventional laparoscopic were performed. There were five conversions from SILS (3.88%) and three conversions from other group (3.95%) to open Kugel or Lichtenstein repairs, but the difference was not significant statistically. The recurrence rate during half year period follow up was 2.3% (3 of 129) for SILS and 1.4% (1 of 76) for conventional one. The chronic pain rate was 4.7% for SILS and 5.2% for other group. Both groups reported only one wound infection. Incisional hernia was rare (only one) in the SILS arm of the study, which occurred at the site of an umbilical hernia. There was no widely difference between the two cohorts in complication rate [31].

A systematic review by Sajid et al. analyzed from 15 comparative studies on 1651 patients evaluating the surgical outcomes of inguinal hernia repair using SILS versus conventional laparoscopic techniques. Recovery time after the surgery was significantly more rapid in SILS compared to the other procedure. Nonetheless, from the perspective of length of hospital stay, operative time both for unilateral and bilateral hernias, post-operative pain score, one-week pain score, hernia recurrence conversion and post-operative complications between two approaches showed an equality. The sub-group analysis of four included randomized, controlled trials showed similarities between outcomes following SILS and conventional laparoscopic procedure except slightly higher postoperative pain score in conventional group [27].

SILS inguinal hernia repair offers better cosmetic results with slightly longer operative time compared to conventional laparoscopic inguinal hernia repair. However, this approach is technically demanding and should be reserved for experienced single incision hernia surgeons [32]. The invention of new surgical tools will hopefully overcome the current obstacles in SILS in the future [27].

## 3. Complication of laparoscopic hernia repair

Even the complications in endoscopic inguinal hernia surgery are more dangerous and more frequent compared to those in open surgery; they could be avoided especially in experienced hands [33]. The complication rate for laparoscopic repair of inguinal hernia ranges from less than 3% to as high as 20% [34].

Complications and the various precautions to be taken in hernia surgery can be divided into:

1. Preoperative

2. Intraoperative

3. Postoperative

### 3.1 Preoperative precautions

Patient with large hernias, obese patients and irreducible, obstructed hernias are best avoided. Strangulated hernia is an absolute contraindication. Elderly patients require a detailed work-up to assess cardiorespiratory status to ensure a safe outcome.

## 3.2 Intraoperative complication

### *3.2.1 Vascular injury*

The iliac vessels, inferior epigastric vessels, spermatic vessels, muscular branches, vessels over the pubic arch (including corona mortis vein) or other vessels in the region are susceptible to injury [33].

### *3.2.2 Visceral injury*

The most common injury occurs is bladder injury. Emptying the bladder prior to an inguinal hernia repair is a must to prevent a trocar injury. It is desirable to catheterize the bladder. When urine is seen in the extraperitoneal space then the diagnosis of this bladder injury is evident. Repair with vicryl in two layers and insert a urinary catheter for 7–10 days are recommended [33].

Bowel injuries take place when trocar insertion or while dissecting hernia or utilizing an electrodiathermy. The incidence of bowel injuries is greatly reduced, but sadly not completely eliminated [35].

### *3.2.3 Pneumoperitoneum*

It is a common occurrence in TEP. The patient is placed in Trendelenburg position and escalating the insufflation pressures to 15 mmHg helps. Insertion of a Veress needle at Palmer's point can be used if the problem still persists [33].

### *3.2.4 Nerve injuries*

There are several nerves, viz., ilioinguinal nerve, iliohypogastric nerve, genito-femoral nerve with its medial and lateral branches (external spermatic nerve and lumboinguinal nerve) which are coursing in the myopectineal orifice of Fruchaud. These are prone to injury especially when a lateral dissection or mesh fixation is being performed. Patient might be suffering from a long-term pain and discomfort [36].

### *3.2.5 Injury to cord structures*

The cord structures might be harmed while dissecting the hernial sac from it. It leads to an eventual fibrotic narrowing of the vas. In a young patient, a complete transection of the vas needs to be done. Finding the vas before releasing any structure near the deep ring or floor of the extraperitoneal space can help to avoid this injury. It should be done gentle and direct and not grasping vas deferens with forceps [33].

### *3.2.6 Bowel obstruction*

A water-tight peritoneal closure should reduce the risk of postoperative intestinal obstruction. Laparoscopy is the procedure of choice to diagnose and treat this complication [37].

A risk reduction strategy is required to improve the clinical outcome and this must be adopted during the following surgical steps:

1. Placement of the trocar and working port

Identify and repair a pneumoperitoneum as a result of reckless insertion of the first trocar. If there any previous surgical scarring, a surgeon must be more attentive and alert in placing the trocar [33, 38].

The underlying intraperitoneal organs like bowel and bladder should not be damaged in trocar insertion process. In midline area, beware of the inferior epigastric vessels which cause copious bleeding. A laparotomy conversion might be considered if any visceral injury is found [39].

2. Dissection of the hernial sac

Identifying the correct anatomical landmarks is the next most decisive step, which is difficult for beginners. The first point is to recognize the pubic bone. After this, the rest of the landmarks can be discovered by putting this as reference point. Keep away the triangle of doom, which contains the iliac vessels and do not place tacks in the triangle of pain laterally [33, 39].

3. Mesh placement and fixation

Choose the appropriate size of the mesh to prevent a later recurrence due to an eventual "shrinkage" of the prosthesis [40]. Slashing the mesh is hindered because it can lead to a recurrence [33].

Several studies have recommended no fixation but have been found wanting. Tissue glues are being used to secure the mesh in place [39, 41, 42].

### 3.3 Post-operative complication

#### *3.3.1 Seroma/hematoma formation*

It is a common complication after laparoscopic hernia surgery and the incidence is within 5–25%. It resolves spontaneously around 4–6 weeks. A drain can be considered if there is an excessive bleeding or after extensive dissection [33].

#### *3.3.2 Urinary retention*

The reported incidence for this complication is 1.3–5.8%, usually found in elderly patients with prostatism. Put a catheter before the surgery and remove the next day morning [33, 43, 44].

#### *3.3.3 Neuralgias*

The incidence is reported to be between 0.5 and 4.6% and intra peritoneal onlay mesh had the highest incidence [43]. The most commonly involved nerves are lateral cutaneous nerve of thigh, genitofemoral nerve and intermediate cutaneous nerve of thigh. This complication can be prevented by avoiding fixing the mesh lateral to the deep inguinal ring in the region of the triangle of pain, safe dissection of a large hernial sac and no dissection of fascia over the psoas [33].

#### *3.3.4 Testicular pain and swelling*

Reported incidence is of 0.9–1.5%. Most are short-term. Orchitis was found occasionally but testicular atrophy was not a complication [33, 43, 44].

*3.3.5 Mesh infection and wound infection*

Wound infection rates are very low. Mesh infection is a very serious complication and care must be taken to maintain strict aseptic precautions during the entire procedure [33].

*3.3.6 Recurrence*

The risk of the need for repair for recurrent hernia following these initial hernia operations was lower for patients with open mesh repair and for patients with laparoscopic mesh repair [33, 45].

Laparoscopic has advantages in treating recurrent inguinal hernia including elimination of the missed hernia, identify a complex hernias, covering entire myopectineal orifice with mesh that buttressing the intrinsic collagen deficit so one of the cause of recurrent hernia could be overcome [14].

## 4. Conclusion

Laparoscopic inguinal hernia repair shows more benefits compared to open hernia repair. SILS inguinal hernia repair offers better cosmetic results; post-operative recovery time was significantly quicker and less painful. However, this approach is technically demanding and should be reserved for experienced single incision hernia surgeons. The invention of new surgical tools will hopefully overcome the current obstacles in SILS in the future.

## Acknowledgements

We would also like to show our gratitude to the Grace Ika Yuwono of Western Sydney University for writing assistance and language editing.

## Conflict of interest

The authors declare no conflict of interest.

## Appendices and nomenclature

| | |
|---|---|
| SILS | single incision laparoscopic surgery |
| TAPP | trans-abdominal pre-peritoneal |
| TEP | totally extra peritoneal |
| CDC | The Centers for Disease Control |

## Author details

Reno Rudiman[1] and Andika August Winata[2*]

1 Director of Digestive Surgery Department, Padjadjaran University, Bandung, West Java, Indonesia

2 General Surgeon in Eka Hospital BSD, Indonesia

*Address all correspondence to: andhika.august@gmail.com

## References


[1] Dindo D, Demartines N, Clavien PA. Classification of surgical complications: A new proposal with evaluation in a cohort of 6336 patients and results of a survey. Annals of Surgery. 2004;**240**(2):205-213

[2] Azoury S, Farrow N, Hu Q, Soares K, Hicks C. Postoperative abdominal wound infection - epidemiology, risk factors, identification, and management. Chronic Wound Care Management and Research. 2015;**2**:137-148

[3] Vecchio R, MacFayden BV, Palazzo F. History of laparoscopic surgery. Panminerva Medica. 2000;**42**(1):87-90

[4] Haribhakti SP, Mistry JH. Techniques of laparoscopic cholecystectomy: Nomenclature and selection. Journal of Minimal Access Surgery. 2015;**11**(2):113-118

[5] Bruhat MA, Chapron C, Mage G, Pouly JL, Canis M, Wattiez A, et al. The benefits and risks of laparoscopic surgery. Revue Française de Gynécologie et d'Obstétrique. 1993;**88**(2):84-88

[6] Agha R, Muir G. Does laparoscopic surgery spell the end of the open surgeon? Journal of the Royal Society of Medicine. 2003;**96**(11):544-546

[7] Khwaja HA, Bonanomi G. Bariatric surgery: Techniques, outcomes and complications. Current Anaesthesia and Critical Care. 2010;**21**(1):31-38

[8] McCormack K, Scott NW, Go PM, Ross S, Grant A, Collaboration the EU HerniaTrialists. Laparoscopic techniques versus open techniques for inguinal hernia repair. Cochrane Database of Systematic Reviews. 2003;(1):Cd001785. DOI: 10.1002/14651858

[9] Reichenbach DJ, Tackett AD, Harris J, Camacho D, Graviss EA, Dewan B, et al. Laparoscopic colon resection early in the learning curve: What is the appropriate setting? Annals of Surgery. 2006;**243**(6):730-737

[10] Budzynski A, Matlok M, Pedziwiatr M, Budzynski P, Tusinski M, Zub-Pokrowiecka A, et al. SILS (single incision laparoscopic surgery) - new surgical approach to peritoneal cavity. Advances in Medical Sciences. 2011;**56**(1):18-24

[11] Froghi F, Sodergren MH, Darzi A, Paraskeva P. Single-incision laparoscopic surgery (SILS) in general surgery: A review of current practice. Surgical Laparoscopy, Endoscopy & Percutaneous Techniques. 2010;**20**(4):191-204

[12] Zinner MJ, Ashley SW. Maingot's Abdominal Operation. 12th edition. New York: Mc Graw-Hill; 2013

[13] Bracale U, Melillo P, Pignata G, Di Salvo E, Rovani M, Merola G, et al. Which is the best laparoscopic approach for inguinal hernia repair: TEP or TAPP? A systematic review of the literature with a network meta-analysis. Surgical Endoscopy. 2012 Dec;**26**(12):3355-3366

[14] de Beaux AC. Abdominal Hernias in Core Topics in General & Emergency Surgery - E-Book: A Companion to Specialist Surgical Practice. Edisi Ke-6th. London: Elsevier Health Sciences; 2018. pp. 81-93. hlm

[15] Lal P, Kajla RK, Chander J, Ramteke VK. Laparoscopic total extraperitoneal (TEP) inguinal hernia repair: Overcoming the learning curve. Surgical Endoscopy. 2004;**18**(4):642-645

[16] Loureiro MP, Trauczynski P, Claus C, Carvalho G, Bonin E, Cavazzola L. Totally Extraperitoneal endoscopic inguinal hernia repair using mini instruments:

Pushing the boundaries of minimally invasive hernia surgery. Journal of Minimally Invasive Surgical Sciences. 2013;**2**(3):8-12

[17] Köckerling F, Bittner R, Jacob DA, Seidelmann L, Keller T, Adolf D, et al. TEP versus TAPP: Comparison of the perioperative outcome in 17,587 patients with a primary unilateral inguinal. Hernia. Surgical Endoscopy. 2015;**29**(12):3750-3760

[18] Rambhia SU, Modi R. A comparative study between totally extraperitoneal and transabdominal preperitoneal laparoscopic inguinal hernia repair techniques. International Surgery Journal. 2017;**4**(2):663-670

[19] Tran HM, Tran K, Zajkowska M, Lam V, Hawthorne W. Single-incision laparoscopic intraperitoneal onlay mesh repair for the treatment of multiple recurrent inguinal hernias. JSLS: Journal of the Society of Laparoendoscopic Surgeons. 2014;**18**(3):1-8

[20] Yussra Y, Sutton PA, Kosai NR, Razman J, Mishra RK, Harunarashid H, et al. Single incision laparoscopic surgery (SILS) inguinal hernia repair - recent clinical experiences of this novel technique. La Clinica Terapeutica. 2013;**164**(5):425-428

[21] Daniel Sánchez López J, Garijo Alvarez J, Garcia-Sancho L, Sánchez-Cabezudo Noguera F, Torres Jiménez J. Single incision laparoscopic surgery (SILS) for incarcerated incisional hernia: A new approach. Cirugía Espanōla. 2009;**88**(3):199-200

[22] Yussra Y, A Sutton P, Kosai NR, Jarmin R, K Mishra R, harunarrashid H, et al. Single incision laparoscopic surgery (SILS) inguinal hernia repair-recent clinical experiences of this novel technique. La Clinica Terapeutica. 2013;**164**(5):425-428

[23] Hirano D, Minei S, Yamaguchi K, Yoshikawa T, Hachiya T, Yoshida T, et al. Retroperitoneoscopic adrenalectomy for adrenal tumors via a single large port. Journal of Endourology. 2005 Sep;**19**(7):788-792

[24] Greaves N, Nicholson J. Single incision laparoscopic surgery in general surgery: A review. Annals of the Royal College of Surgeons of England. 2011;**93**(6):437-440

[25] Petter-Puchner AH, Brunner W, Gruber-Blum S, Glaser KS, Fortelny R. A systematic review of hernia surgery in SIL (single-incision laparoscopy) technique. European Surgery. 2014;**46**(3):113-117

[26] Rajapandian S, Bhushan C, Sabnis SC, Jain M, Raj PP, Parathasarthi R, et al. Single incision multiport versus conventional laparoscopic inguinal hernia repair: A matched comparison. Journal of Minimal Access Surgery. 2018;**14**(1):44-51

[27] Sajid MS, Khawaja AH, Sayegh M, Baig MK. A systematic review comparing single-incision versus multi-incision laparoscopic surgery for inguinal hernia repair with mesh. International Journal of Surgery. 2016;**29**:25-35

[28] Vidal O, Valentini M, Ginesta C, Marti J, Espert JJ, Benarroch G, et al. Laparoendoscopic single-site surgery appendectomy. Surgical Endoscopy. 2010 Mar;**24**(3):686-691

[29] Ece I, Yilmaz H, Yormaz S, Shahin M. Clinical outcomes of single incision laparoscopic surgery and conventional laparoscopic transabdominal preperitoneal inguinal hernia repair. Journal of Minimal Access Surgery. 2017;**13**:37-41

[30] Tran H. Safety and efficacy of single incision laparoscopic surgery for total extraperitoneal inguinal hernia repair. JSLS: Journal of the Society of Laparoendoscopic Surgeons. 2011;**15**(1):47-52

[31] Buckley FP 3rd, Vassaur H, Monsivais S, Sharp NE, Jupiter D, Watson R, et al. Comparison of outcomes for single-incision laparoscopic inguinal herniorrhaphy and traditional three-port laparoscopic herniorrhaphy at a single institution. Surgical Endoscopy. 2014;**28**(1):30-35

[32] Yang GP, Tung KL. A comparative study of single incision versus conventional laparoscopic inguinal hernia repair. Hernia: The Journal of Hernias and Abdominal Wall Surgery. 2015;**19**(3):401-405

[33] Chowbey PK, Pithawala M, Khullar R, Sharma A, Soni V, Baijal M. Complications in groin hernia surgery and the way out. Journal of Minimal Access Surgery. 2006;**2**(3):174-177

[34] Johansson B, Hallerback B, Glise H, Anesten B, Smedberg S, Roman J. Laparoscopic mesh versus open preperitoneal mesh versus conventional technique for inguinal hernia repair: A randomized multicenter trial (SCUR hernia repair study). Annals of Surgery. 1999;**230**(2):225-231

[35] Felix EL, Harbertson N, Vartanian S. Laparoscopic hernioplasty: Significant complications. Surgical Endoscopy. 1999;**13**(4):328-331

[36] Kraus MA. Nerve injury during laparoscopic inguinal hernia repair. Surgical Laparoscopy and Endoscopy. 1993;**3**(4):342-345

[37] Cueto J, Vázquez JA, Solís MA, Valdéz G, Valencia S, Weber A. Bowel obstruction in the postoperative period of laparoscopic inguinal hernia repair (TAPP): Review of the literature. JSLS: Journal of the Society of Laparoendoscopic Surgeons. 1998;**2**(3):277-280

[38] Dulucq JL, Wintringer P, Mahajna A. Totally extraperitoneal (TEP) hernia repair after radical prostatectomy or previous lower abdominal surgery: Is it safe? A prospective study. Surgical endoscopy. 2006;**20**(3):473-476

[39] Lomanto D, AN K. Managing intra-operative complications during totally extraperitoneal repair of inguinal hernia. Journal of Minimal Access Surgery. 2006;**2**:165-170

[40] Schumpelick V, Klinge U, Welty G, Klosterhalfen B. Meshes within the abdominal wall. Der Chirurg; Zeitschrift fur alle Gebiete der operativen Medizen. 1999;**70**(8):876-887

[41] Ferzli GS, Frezza EE, Pecoraro AM Jr, Ahern KD. Prospective randomized study of stapled versus unstapled mesh in a laparoscopic preperitoneal inguinal hernia repair. Journal of the American College of Surgeons. 1999;**188**(5):461-465

[42] Smith AI, Royston CM, Sedman PC. Stapled and nonstapled laparoscopic transabdominal preperitoneal (TAPP) inguinal hernia repair. A prospective randomized trial. Surgical Endoscopy. 1999;**13**(8):804-806

[43] Fitzgibbons RJ Jr, Camps J, Cornet DA, Nguyen NX, Litke BS, Annibali R, et al. Laparoscopic inguinal herniorrhaphy. Results of a multicenter trial. Annals of Surgery. 1995;**221**(1):3-13

[44] Phillips EH, Arregui M, Carroll BJ, Corbitt J, Crafton WB, Fallas MJ, et al. Incidence of complications following laparoscopic hernioplasty. Surgical Endoscopy. 1995;**9**(1):16-21

[45] Kokotovic D, Bisgaard T, Helgstrand F. Long-term recurrence and complications associated with elective incisional hernia repair. Journal of the American Medical Association. 2016;**316**(15):1575-1582

Section 4

# Rare Hernias

Chapter 9

# Rare Presentations of Hernia

*Ashanga Yatawatta*

## Abstract

Rare types of hernias require the use of astute clinical judgment and high index of suspicion with supportive information obtained with cross sectional imaging. Having a clear understanding is important to the current surgeon as well as gynecologist. This chapter attempts to compile the common types of these rare hernias to discuss anatomical defects, imaging features and treatment options. Technical details of treatment are not offered for each type in detail due to limited scope of this text. The emphasis on clinical examination and judgment cannot be overstated and depending on cross sectional imaging alone for clinical diagnosis is discouraged. Introduction of minimally invasive surgery has changed the landscape for rare hernias with some new types being added—such as port site hernia—but mostly with less invasive treatment options being added to the armament. It is expected that laparoscopic hernia repair for these rare hernias will be soon the preferred modality of treatment.

**Keywords:** spigelian hernia, obturator hernia, Richter hernia, Amyand hernia, De Garengeot hernia, Littre hernia, reduction en-masse of hernia, interparietal hernia, sciatic hernia, perineal hernia, parastomal hernia

## 1. Introduction

Hernia surgery is one the commonest procedure performed today. Although the vast majority of hernias are typical on presentation, there are rare types, which can confuse even the most experienced surgeons [1]. Having an understanding behind the anatomy, appearance on imaging and treatment principles are important for the contemporary surgeon, as the likelihood of coming across one would be the limiting factor during an average career [2]. Clinical features of each type tend to be subtle and frequently overlapping, therefore a clear understanding of clinical features as well as supporting imaging information in critical for accurate diagnosis and treatment planning. Important surgical history is embedded with most of these rare hernias as all of these were recognized, treated, and taught clinically in an era with no supporting imaging facilities.

## 2. Spigelian hernia

Spigelian hernia occurs due to a weakness of the spigelian fascia, which is the layer between rectus muscle and semilunar line [3]. The absence of a posterior rectus sheath is a contributing factor at this location and therefore mostly occurs below the arcuate line. Most of these are smaller than 2 cm and clinical findings may be obscured by the intact anterior rectus sheath, giving rise to the impression of no hernia being present [4]. Astute clinical judgment is needed with confirmation by CT or ultrasound on an elderly patient with atypical pain and tenderness on the typical location, as the presence of a lump may not always be associated [5].

The risk of incarceration and strangulation is high due to the small neck and lack of clinical features to suspect as such. Incidentally discovered spigelian hernia is treated aggressively to minimize this risk unlike most other inguinal hernia's, which can be observed. Traditional open anatomical repair consists of open reduction of hernia and closure of overlying muscles along the lines of least tension, but laparoscopic mesh repair offers a more simple and durable option [6]. Laparoscopic and Robotic surgery port placement of more than 10 mm size can also increase the risk of spigelian hernia, especially an angled trajectory in the subcutaneous tissues with fascial weakness not directly overlying the skin incision.

## 3. Obturator hernia

Obturator hernia occurs through the osseous defect bounded by pubic bone and ischium, usually covered by a membrane with fenestrations for the obturator neurovascular bundle. Weakening of the membrane leads to enlargement of this defect, leading to formation of a hernia [7]. Weight loss and pelvic side wall muscle wasting are associated, but lack of exam findings makes the diagnosis difficult. Howship-Romberg sign results from compression of the obturator nerve by hip flexion but current diagnosis is mostly aided by CT.

Open exploration is usually needed due to the partial of complete bowel obstruction usually associated with the presentation [8]. Complete reduction of the hernia sac and contents is performed and preperitoneal fat pad found within the obturator canal needs to be reduced, oftentimes requiring manipulation of the nerve with a nerve hook. The defined margin of the defect is covered with prosthetic mesh. The place of laparoscopy is usually limited to non-emergent situations and follows the same principles as open repair [9].

## 4. Lumbar hernia

Two different types are encountered according to the anatomy. Superior lumbar triangle is bounded by 12th rib, paraspinal muscles, and the internal oblique muscles (Grynfeltt's triangle) While the Inferior lumbar triangle, which is bounded by the Iliac crest, latissimus dorsi muscle, and external oblique muscle leads to Petit's triangle hernia [10, 11]. The overlapping nature of bulky muscles prevent the usual occurrence of hernias in these locations but acquired weakness after surgery, especially muscle cutting incisions or nerve damage leads to protrusion of lumbar fascia with extraperitoneal fat and an occasional hernial sac. The large defect makes incarceration difficult, but patient may complain of back pain, cosmesis, or weakness of activities associated with use of these muscles, in addition to the presence of a visible lump. CT is essential to diagnose especially with a prior incision to exclude incisional hernia [12].

Treatment is limited due to fixed bony landmarks anchoring muscle and large overlapping mesh repairs offers the best options. Both open and laparoscopic options are available but open repair adds the risk of further muscle weakness or nerve damage in addition to wound complications [13].

## 5. Richter's hernia

Richter's hernia occurs when part of the circumference of the intestinal wall is contained in a hernia sac, most commonly incarcerated. This can progress to strangulation but typically will not demonstrate obstructive features due to patency of part of the lumen [14]. This atypical feature leads to high rates of missing the diagnosis, even among experienced surgeons. Common anatomical sites include femoral and indirect inguinal hernias and of increasing frequency in the laparoscopic era, port site hernias.

Careful clinical examination might allow discovery of the tender lump at the common sites but mostly needs confirmation with CT.

Treatment depends on the degree of ischemic insult to the bowel wall. Laparoscopic assessment would be appropriate with viable bowel being reduced and mesh repair being optimal. However, any concerns for strangulation would need open exploration for bowel assessment, resection if necessary and anatomical repair of the hernia. An exception would be early port site hernia after laparoscopic surgery, where anatomical repair with non-absorbable sutures would be appropriate for a defect less than 2 cm [15].

## 6. Amyand's hernia

Amyand's hernia describes the presence of appendix within the hernia sac and typically found at surgery for inguinal hernia [16, 17]. The appendix may or may not be inflamed at time of surgery and treatment differs accordingly. Although typical Amyand's hernia are described for inguinal hernia, it is likely to be found in any viscera containing sac, but only femoral hernias are given a different name, as De Garengeot's hernia.

Treatment of non-inflamed appendix found at time of hernia surgery does not include appendectomy for two reasons. Appendectomy in not indicated and subsequent episodes of appendicitis can easily be confirmed by CT and laparoscopically treated, which is different when only open surgery was the surgical option. In addition, placing prosthetic mesh increases the risk of infection after breaching intestinal lumen. Therefore, incidentally found appendix could be left alone and hernia repair performed as indicated, mostly with mesh placement [18].

The presence of inflamed appendix changes this approach significantly. Appendectomy and source control of sepsis is paramount for a good outcome. If the incision for hernia is not appropriate, a suitable incision is beneficial for safe access. A midline incision will also allow closure of weakened area of the posterior wall with absorbable sutures from within and allow an interval hernia repair with mesh. Use of prosthetic mesh is discourage although some have shown acceptable results with absorbable or biological mesh placement.

In the modern era of high-quality cross-sectional imaging, surprises in the OR should be the exception rather than the rule. Therefore, proper planning and informed consent should be carried out before heading to the OR. This would still allow surgeons to offer treatment options from a laparoscopic approach, especially for bilateral hernia.

## 7. De Garengeot's hernia

The presence of appendix in the femoral hernia sac is rare and follows the same principles as for Amyand's hernia [19, 20]. Femoral hernia, having less content compared with an inguinal hernia, makes finding an appendix even more remote. However, recurrences for femoral hernia are much less without use of prosthetic mesh and therefore, in the appropriate clinical setting, a combined appendectomy and femoral hernia repair would be having less long-term complications [21].

## 8. Littre's hernia

The unusual presence of a Meckel's diverticulum in a hernia sac is described as a Littre's hernia. This hernia is inguinal in half of cases and umbilical or femoral in the other half [22, 23]. The presence of ileum attached to the diverticulum is not unusual in addition to the persistent omphalo-mesenteric tract. Inflammation of the diverticulum at time of hernia surgery in highly unusual and according to current surgical principles, non-inflamed diverticula are not resected during incidental discovery, unless in a child. Diverticulitis and less frequent perforation need resection and source control and hernia repair has to be limited to anatomical repair or biological mesh placement, with resultant high recurrence rates. A safer alternative would be to defer the hernia repair with prosthetic mesh for a later date and treat the diverticulum alone. Depending on experience and technical expertise, an argument could be made for either of these procedures as laparoscopic procedures, in select cases [24].

## 9. Reduction en-masse

Attempts at aggressive reduction of incarcerated hernia can lead to false "reduction" at skin level but intestine loops being still trapped within a no yielding fascial "neck" and can lead to persistent incarceration and strangulation. Implications of these late complications are devastating due to failure to recognize early and uncontained leakage leading to widespread peritonitis, unlike local peritonitis within the hernia sac.

Inguinal hernia is the commonest type complicated by reduction en-masse, as the first treatment option at initial presentation with incarceration seems to be attempted reduction. Health economics have forced emergency room visits to be kept brief and this might have made this option more popular, as the expected enthusiasm for emergency surgery for incarceration is less than the eagerness of ER providers in testing "their method of reduction". A recent review suggests to observe the patient overnight in ER, following reduction for possible reduction en-masse and offer elective surgery within a reasonable time period afterward [25].

## 10. Interparietal hernia

This rare hernia type occurs due to a fascial defect leading to the hernia sac being positioned within the layers of the abdominal wall. It may be considered as a hernia in evolution but not showing protrusion through the skin. These hernias are mostly associated with incisions and port site hernias, are an example. Richter type hernia and spigelian hernia are strongly associated with interparietal hernia type [26].

Clinical features are not typical, and diagnosis is based off cross sectional imaging. Diagnostic laparoscopy in invasive for diagnosis but can be combined with treatment at same setting. Smaller fascial defects—typically less than 2 cm—may show good results with anatomical repair but larger hernias will need mesh placement. Laparoscopic mesh repair is mostly appropriate but in the presence of questionable bowel viability, an open repair and bowel resection might need to be combined with a component separation technique to bridge the defect [27].

## 11. Sciatic hernia

The greater sciatic foramen can accommodate a hernia sac for unclear reasons. These are extremely uncommon and frequently asymptomatic until obstruction becomes the first symptom. A tender lump may be felt on the gluteal region, but cross-sectional imaging is crucial for correct diagnosis. Sciatic nerve irritation by the pressure is an unusual presentation [28].

Treatment is exploration via laparotomy in the presence of questionable viability of bowel. Reduction can be achieved with gently traction but attention to sciatic nerve will be crucial to prevent complications. Prosthetic mesh placement is usually preferred. An unusual method of transgluteal approach has been described but this needs very clear diagnosis and positive information about the viability of bowel before commitment [29].

## 12. Perineal hernia

Loss of muscle tone of the pelvic diaphragm leads to weakness and descent of viscera through the perineum. This is rare and typically associated with acquired defects as well congenital abnormalities. Common surgeries associated include abdominoperineal resection, vaginal hysterectomy, and perineal prostatectomy. Multiple vaginal deliveries—especially with difficult, prolonged labor—can lead to primary perineal hernias in older women and these can be quite large in size. An important distinction from utero-vaginal prolapse or rectal prolapse needs clinical acumen and cross-sectional imaging [30].

Treatment approach is transabdominal with some cases needing additional trans-perineal approach as well. Principles remain the same with reduction of hernia sac, inspecting contents to confirm viable bowel and repair with mesh. The bony pelvis is used to anchor the mesh and similarities of treatment of diaphragmatic hernia are seen in treatment of perineal hernia with the types of mesh and anchoring methods. Anatomical repairs are suggested for small hernias but due to primary pathology remaining at large, recurrences are expected to be high [31].

## 13. Parastomal hernia

Parastomal hernias are part of the process in creating any stoma. The defect in the muscular layer is needed for the bowel to be positioned without undue tension or risk to blood supply but larger than necessary space or widening space with time, will allow the additional room to be used for visceral herniation. The principles of muscle splitting and cruciate incisions on the fascia can only minimize this risk [32].

A surprisingly 50% of colostomies will result in a parastomal hernia. However, due to the laxity at the neck, the vast majority remain asymptomatic and treatment is only recommended when ostomy function is impaired or due to cosmetic concerns. Part of this reluctance is due to same risk remaining with the treatment of the parastomal hernia.

The treatment options include primary fascial repair, prosthetic repair, and stoma relocation [33, 34]. The least complex of these options would be fascial repair with a peri-stomal incision, but this carries a high recurrence rate. The only advantage is avoidance of entering the peritoneal cavity. This surgery is recommended for patient at high risk for a laparotomy, but a better option would be nonintervention rather than increasing the risk of a procedure with a high recurrence rate.

Relocation may be an option but requires a laparotomy and carries hernia formation at previous site as well as new site. Use of mesh would be one way to minimize this risk, but other complications associated with erosion, infection, and obstruction are important to consider in the decision making. The least risk of recurrence is with use of prosthetic mesh but the complications of placing a permanent foreign body next to bowel carries significant risks by itself. The method of mesh placement can be laparoscopic or open and can be placed onlay, retro-rectus or intra-abdominally. The Sugarbaker method of placing the mesh against the wall, creating a long angulated tunnel for the bowel to exit, seems to be one of the simplest methods when done as a laparoscopic procedure. However, many methods have been described with excellent results and no method is inferior, as long as basic surgical principles are followed.

**Author details**

Ashanga Yatawatta[1,2]

1 Duke LifePoint Health System, Tennessee, United States

2 SurgTech Surgical Solutions LLC, Las Vegas, United States

*Address all correspondence to: ayatawatta@gmail.com

## References

[1] The HerniaSurger Group. International guidelines for groin hernia management. Hernia. 2018;**22**:1-165

[2] Simons MP, Aufenacker T, Bay-Nielsen M, et al. European hernia society guidelines on the treatment of intuinal hernia in adult patients. Hernia. 2009;**13**:343-403

[3] Rankin A, Kostusiak M, Sokker A. Spigelian hernia: Case series and review of the literature. Visceral Medicine. 2019;**35**(2):133-136

[4] Pinna A, Cossu ML, Paliogiannis P, et al. Spigelian hernia: A series of cases and literature review. Annali Italiani di Chirurgia. 2016;**87**:306-311

[5] Alfonzo M et al. Point of care ultrasound identification of an abdominal hernia. Pediatric Emergency Care. 2017;**33**(8):596-598

[6] Barnes TG, McWhinnie DL. Laparoscopic spigelian hernia repair: A systemic review. Surgical Laparoscopy, Endoscopy & Percutaneous Techniques. 2016;**26**(4):265-270

[7] Drokas DD et al. Radiographic and surgical findings of type 1 obturator hernias in patients with refractory groin pain. Clinical Imaging. 2019;**55**:35-40

[8] Sa NC, Silva VCM, et al. Rare case of incarcerated obturator hernia: Case report and review of literature. International Journal of Surgery Case Reports. 2017;**37**:157-160

[9] Caine EA, Newman TH, et al. Subacute bowel obstruction secondary to an obturator hernia: case report and a review of the literature. Journal of Surgical Case Reports. 2017;**2017**(4):rjx061

[10] Piozzi GN et al. Management criteria of Grynfeltt's lumbar hernia: A case report and review of literature. Cureus. 2019;**11**(1):e3865

[11] Graulas A, Lallemand B, Krick M. The retroperitoneoscopic repair of a lumbar hernia of petit. Case report and review of literature. Acta Chirurgica Belgica. 2004;**104**(3):330-334

[12] Martin J et al. MDCT of abdominal wall lumbar hernias: anatomical review, pathological findings and differential diagnosis. Surgical and Radiologic Anatomy. 2012;**34**(5):455-463

[13] Capasso L et al. Primary acquired Grynfeltt hernia: two new cases and literature review. Annali Italiani di Chirurgia. 2018;**89**:255-260

[14] Foster D, Nagarajan S, Panait L. Richter-type spigelian hernia: A case report and review of the literature. International Journal of Surgery Case Reports. 2015;**6C**:160-162

[15] Sahsamanis G, Samaras S, Gkouzis K, Dimitrakopoulos G. Strangulated Richter's incisional hernia presenting as an abdominal mass with necrosis of the overlapping skin. A case report and review of the literature. Clinical Case Reports. 30 Jan 2017;**5**(3):253-256. DOI: 10.1002/ccr3.776

[16] Kromka W, Rau AS, Fox CJ. Amyand's hernia with acute gangrenous appendicitis and cecal perforation. A case report and review of the literature. International Journal of Surgery Case Reports. 2018;**44**:8-10

[17] Shaban Y et al. Amyand's hernia: A case report and review of the literature. International Journal of Case Reports. 2018;**47**:92-96

[18] Holmes K, Guinn JE. Amyand hernia repair with mesh and

appendectomy. Surgical Case Reports. 2019;**5**(1):42

[19] O'Connor A, Asaad P. De Garengeot's hernia with appendicitis – a rare cause of acutely painful groin swelling. Journal of Surgical Case Reports. 2019;**2019**(5):rjz142

[20] Bidarmarghz B, Borrowdale RC, Raufian K. A rare presentation of appendicitis inside the femoral canal: Case report and literature review. Surgical Case Reports. 2018;**4**(1):143

[21] Linder S, Linder G, Mansson C. Treatment of de Garengeot's hernia. A meta analysis. Hernia. 2019;**23**(1):131-141

[22] Schizas D et al. Littre's hernia: A systemic review of the literature. Hernia. 2019;**23**(1):125-130

[23] Pampal A, Aksakal ED. Littre hernia in childhood: a case report with a brief review of the literature. African Journal of Paediatric Surgery. 2011;**8**(2):221-224

[24] Skandalakis PN, Zoras O, Skandalakis JE, Mirilas P. Littre hernia: surgical anatomy, embryology and technique of repair. The American Surgeon. 2006;**72**(3):238-243. Review

[25] Yatawatta A. Reduction en-masse of inguinal hernia: A review of a rare and potential fatal complication following reduction of inguinal hernia. Case Reports. 2017;**2017**:bcr-2017-220475

[26] Davis JR et al. Interparietal hernia complicating retromuscular ventral hernia repair. The American Surgeon. 2016;**82**(7):658-659

[27] Sakamoto T et al. Laparoscopic reduction and repair of a strangulated interparietal inguinal hernia. Asian Journal of Endoscopic Surgery. 2016;**9**(1):83-85

[28] Karasaki T, Nakagawa T, Tanaka N. Sciatic hernia: Is it really rare? Surgery Today. 2014;**44**(6):1079-1083

[29] Losanoff JE, Basson MD, Gruber SA, Weaver DW. Sciatic hernia: A comprehensive review of the world literature (1900-2008). American Journal of Surgery. 2010;**199**(1):52-59

[30] Balla A et al. Perineal hernia repair after abdominoperineal excision or extrelevator abdominoperineal excision. A systemic review of the literature. Techniques in Coloproctology. 2017;**21**(5):329-336

[31] Musters GD et al. Is there a place for a biological mesh in perineal hernia repair? Hernia. 2016;**20**(5):747-754

[32] Fox SS et al. An evaluation of parastomal hernia repair using the Americas hernia society quality collaborative. The American Surgeon. 2017;**83**(8):881-886

[33] Chapman SJ, Wood B, Drake TM, Young N, Jayne DG. Systemic review and meta-analysis of prophylactic mesh during primary stoma formation to prevent parastomal hernia. Diseases of the Colon and Rectum. 2017;**60**(1):107-115. review

[34] Antoniou SA et al. European hernia society guidelines on prevention and treatment of parastomal hernias. Hernia. 2018;**22**(1):183-198

Chapter 10

# Laparoscopic Rare Abdominal Hernia Treatment

*Emrah Akin, Baris Mantoglu, Fatih Altintoprak and Necattin Firat*

## Abstract

Diaphragm and abdominal wall hernias are rare, and they may be congenital or acquired. Spiegel hernia incidence is between 0.1 and 2%. Morgagni hernia is comprising only 2–3% of all diaphragmatic hernias. Most Spiegel and Morgagni hernias are diagnosed late because of their non-specific symptoms and asymptomatic clinical presentation. The major symptoms are abdominal pain, vomiting, and dyspnea. Computed tomography (CT) shows the hernia sac content, strangulation or incarceration in the content, and detailed anatomical information about surrounding tissue. Surgery is the main treatment option except patients who have severe comorbidity. Spiegel hernia surgery can be performed open or laparoscopic. Intraperitoneal onlay mesh (IPOM), total extraperitoneal procedure (TEP), transabdominal preperitoneal (TAPP) procedure, or partial transabdominal laparoscopic methods are minimal invasive surgery options. In the repair of Morgagni hernia, surgical options may be laparoscopy, laparotomy, thoracotomy, or thoracoscopy.

**Keywords:** rare abdominal hernias, laparoscopic hernia treatment, Spiegel hernia, Morgagni hernia

## 1. Spiegel hernia

### 1.1 Introduction

Spiegel hernia is a rare congenital or acquired abdominal wall hernia [1]. It is between 0.1 and 2% of all abdominal wall hernias and is one of the diseases that a surgeon can face during his professional life with the frequency of not exceeding the number of fingers of a hand. Transverse abdominis aponeurosis in the area between the semilunar line and the lateral sheath of the rectus is called Spiegel's fascia, and from this point preperitoneal fat tissue or intraabdominal organs protruding are defined as Spiegel hernia (SH) [2]. Ninety percent of hernias occur on the transverse line approximately 6 cm above the interspinous line [3]. It has an increasing frequency with age, peaks in the fifth decade, and is more common in women and left side of the abdominal wall [4]. In the diagnosis, the presence of palpable swelling in the left lower quadrant with Valsalva maneuver is sufficient for surgical decision. Clinical suspicion is important in the absence of a palpable mass.

## 1.2 History

The semilunar line is the medial border of the transverse abdominis muscle in the cranio-caudal extension and was first described by the Belgian anatomist, Adriaan van der Spieghel, in the seventeenth century. Its clinical presence was demonstrated in 1764 by a Belgian anatomist, Josef Klinkosh, and was named after him in honor of Spieghel [5]. The disease, which traditionally underwent open surgical procedures with mesh or non-mesh primarily, has been laparoscopically treated by the first time by Carter and Mites in 1992 [6]. The first laparoscopic extra-abdominal approach was published in 1999 by Moreno-Egea [7]. Nowadays, laparoscopy with intraperitoneal onlay mesh, transabdominal preperitoneal approach, total extraperitoneal approach, and partial extraperitoneal treatment options is applied.

## 1.3 General information

### *1.3.1 Physiopathology*

Musculo-aponeurosis of the transversus abdominis extends in the cranial region from the costa to the inguinal region where the tendon conjugate ends in the caudal direction and its medial edge is called linea semilunaris. The lateral sheath of the rectus muscle also extends from the costal margin to the pubis. The Spiegel fascia is located between these two lines and includes fused transverse abdominis aponeurosis and internal oblique muscle [8]. The arcuate or semicircular line defines the boundary of the posterior sheath of the rectus, and as classical information below this line, three muscular aponeuroses proceed over the rectus sheath. Spiegel's hernia is a defect that occurs in the Spiegel's fascia where transverse abdominis and internal oblique fascia layers have lost their integrity but the external oblique remains intact (**Figure 1**). This information explains why these types of hernias are separated from incisional hernias, the difficulty of detecting them at the physical examination, and the fact that they cannot be detected without opening the external oblique layer during surgery [9].

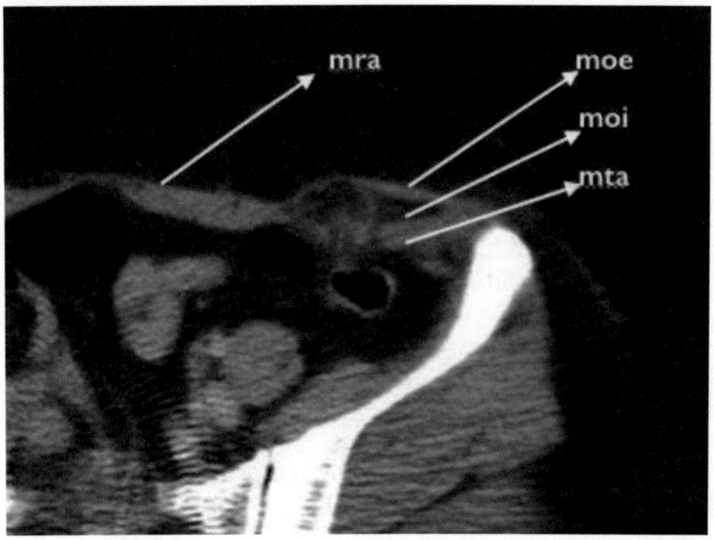


**Figure 1.**
*Spiegel hernia at computerized tomography which consists only two layers of the abdomen wall. moe-musculus obliq externus, moi-musculus obliq internus, mta-musculus transversus abdominis, mra-musculus rectus abdominis.*

There are various theories that this type of abdominal hernias consists of two layers, not all three layers of the abdominal wall. Smaller perforating vascular structures were thought to weaken this anatomy but could not be confirmed by observations. It was also thought that almost a parallel route of internal oblique muscle and transversus abdominis muscle may be another reason. In addition, it has been shown that the frequency of SH below the arcuate line is not a reason for the weakness of the abdominal wall in a structure where all three muscle layers maintain their integrity [1]. The theory has lost its validity with a series of 27 cases in which the patients had herniation above the arcuate line. The disease can be seen congenitally in infants and children as a result of the defect of the mesenchymal layers and is usually associated with increased incidence of cryptorchidism in this age group [10]. On the other hand, the disease is mostly acquired in adults. Pathophysiologically, different series have shown that the disease begins with protruding extraperitoneal fat tissue due to small divisions between the fascia layers. Over time, this small interstitial hernia develops and becomes palpable when it forms the peritoneal sac. This natural course explains the increase in the frequency of the disease with age. Probably hernia presents at any time; reasons that increase intraabdominal pressure are chronic obstructive pulmonary disease (COPD), obesity, chronic constipation, pregnancy, and abnormalities that weaken the abdominal wall including connective tissue diseases and aging which eventually expands the hernia and become symptomatic [11].

#### *1.3.2 Symptomatology and clinical presentation*

Patients usually present with lower abdominal pain and palpable swelling or both. Young patients may have only a small hernia defect with pain, or some may experience swelling with deep palpation. If a palpable mass is present, it may be reduced or not reduced [12]. Typically, the fascia defect is smaller than the sac, and irreductibility is more common, as it is described as a T- or fungus-shaped dead space between internal oblique and external oblique. This phenomenon also explains the tendency to emergency clinical presentation. Obstruction and strangulation rates have been reported between 10 and 29% in different studies and are not uncommon [13, 14].

#### *1.3.3 Diagnosis*

The presence of a palpable mass at the lateral edge of the rectus with increased intraabdominal pressure is sufficient for the diagnosis and surgical decision of SH if there is no previous surgical history. However, in the presence of SH, external oblique fascia or thick fat layer in obese patients may prevent the swelling in physical examination, and at this point clinical suspicion is important in diagnosis. Ultrasonography (USG) as an advanced radiological evaluation may also indicate the size of the fascia defect but is an individual-dependent method. Computed tomography or magnetic resonance imaging (MRI) will be more useful in the evaluation of the hernia content, its relationship with the layers of the abdominal wall, and thus in the selection of the surgical method, but sometimes these tests may also be negative in the absence of palpable swelling. Transperitoneal laparoscopy is useful in both diagnosis and treatment, but it can detect only those with peritoneal sac. Laparoscopic total extraperitoneal method may be appropriate for the detection of hernias containing extraperitoneal fat tissue, which is the most common clinical presentation especially in patients under the age of 50 years, but it is not easy to detect the hernias above the arcuate line for this method, and it is difficult to make TEP decision for each patient with abdominal pain in the lower quadrant [15].

If there is a strong enough suspicion about a small interstitial SH, the diagnosis can be made by open surgery. For asymptomatic patients and those with significant medical comorbidity, surgery is the only effective treatment option because of the high risk of acute clinical presentation.

### *1.3.4 Surgical indication*

The choice of open or laparoscopic surgery is related to the surgeon's experience, the patient's BMI, and the stage of the hernia, according to this:

Stage I: Relatively young patients with a fascia defect below 2 cm. They typically present with well-localized pain and absence of palpable mass. Open surgical method is appropriate in these patients. At surgery, the surgeon may not be able to detect a hernia sac, but exploration should be completed by opening the external oblique fascia and examining all musculofascial layers. Primary repair is often sufficient. In a study of 70 cases published by Larsen and Failey, recurrence was reported as 4.3% in patients treated primarily with open technique [16]. If mesh is to be applied, it can be extraperitoneal or placed in the retromuscular space medially and surrounded by deep planes of the external oblique muscle laterally. In this technique, the frequency of mesh reaction, wound infection, and recurrence is higher.

Stage II: Patients with a fascia defect between 2 and 5 cm and a peritoneal hernia sac. In these patients, the presence of a hernia sac can be palpable or not therewithal hernia contents can be reduced or not. These patients can be operated open or laparoscopically. Small defects can only be closed with laparoscopic primary suture. For larger defects, IPOM, TEP, TAPP, and partial extraperitoneal laparoscopic repair options are available. TEP and TAPP are the techniques of detachment of the peritoneum and repairing of the defect of working extraperitoneal or transperitoneal as similar to inguinal hernia surgery. A MEDLİNE search of the published literature shown that 232 cases in which the results of SH patients operated between 1997 and 2017 were evaluated; the most common choice was IPOM 32%, TEP 30%, and TAPP 22%. In laparoscopic mesh repair, onlay mesh, mesh extended to the retrorectus cavity, mesh repair placed in the extraperitoneal space were defined at the largest case series of 107 cases of laparoscopic repair which was published by Weber et al. [17]. The risk of neurovascular injury in the posterolateral abdominal wall due to the tacker usage for abdominal wall fixation of these meshes is reported to be higher in IPOM and TAPP operations.

Stage III: It is relatively old patients whose facial defects are superior to 5 cm; the integrity of the abdominal wall is mostly deteriorated. The hernia is easily palpable and deductible. In these patients, open surgery is recommended because abdominal wall reconstructions and abdominoplasty may be required. Component separation techniques are not recommended when the hernia is located laterally, but peritoneal flap hernioplasty may be useful. In a series of 22 cases published by Moreno and Egea comparing the results of laparoscopic and open surgery, morbidity and length of stay were significantly higher in the open group, with less pain, less wound infection, and better cosmetic results in the laparoscopic group [7]. In addition, concurrent surgery and wide visualization can be considered as the advantage of laparoscopic approach.

We prefer to perform IPOM technique in our clinic, and herein we will discuss about this technique here. In IPOM, the peritoneal flap is not required, and the surgeon is more familiar with the intraabdominal approach and the advantages of the trocar positioning. However, when selecting mesh type, the surgeon should be careful because of contact with the visceral organs and possible future intraabdominal adhesions. However, to date, no case series of mesh complications have been reported. One patient recurrence has been reported by Kelly et al. after a 40-case series in which laparoscopic intervention was performed [18].

### 1.4 Intraperitoneal onlay mesh technique (IPOM)

#### *1.4.1 Operating room layout*

The patient is placed in the supine position on the operating table with her legs closed. The laparoscopic tower is placed on the right or left side of the patient. The patient's arm opposite the hernia defect is closed. The surgical team settles on the operating table in the opposite direction of the hernia defect. Nasogastric and Foley catheters are placed.

#### *1.4.2 Surgical instruments*

- Standard laparoscopy equipment consisting of a camera, monitor, light, and insufflator.
- 10 mm diameter and 30° angle camera.
- 3 trocar, one 10 mm, 25 mm in diameter.
- Endo Instruments (Atraumatic clamp, dissector, scissors, hook, portegue, aspirator).
- Endo Close®.
- Sealing device with a diameter of –5 mm.
- Composite or dual-coated special-shaped patch according to the size of hernia defect.
- Fixing material for mesh fixation and peritoneal closure (mechanical punch, tissue glue, or nonabsorbable suture material).

#### *1.4.3 Port location selection and surgical technique*

After the patient is stained and covered under sterile conditions under general anesthesia, the abdomen is entered through the right or left upper quadrant distant from the hernia defect with the Hasson technique. After placing the 10 mm trocar and exploring the abdomen, two more 5 mm trocar are inserted under direct vision with transillumination from the farthest point to the hernia defect, making both working ports 90° (**Figure 2**).

The size, localization, and the organs of the hernia defect are evaluated by intraabdominal exploration. The hernia content is evaluated for strangulation or incarceration. After hernia contents are reduced to the abdomen, adhesions are separated by sharp and blunt dissections with energy devices. Even if the hernia sac is visible, it does not need to be removed. Henceforth defect repair is initiated (**Figure 3**).

After suturing the cranial and caudal edges of the mesh with polyprolene to composite or dual mesh, which is suitable for hernia sac size, than introduced through the abdomen from 10 mm port. With the help of Endo Close®, which is inserted through the 2 mm incisions from the outside of the abdomen at the points

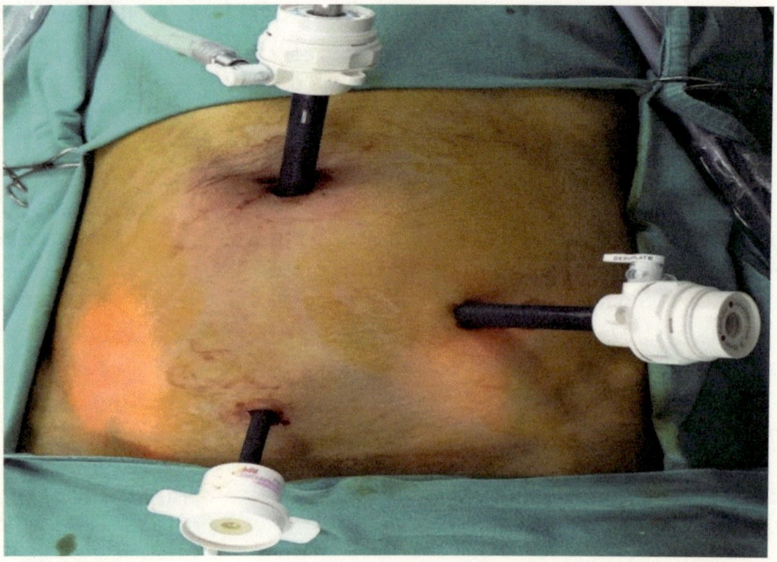

**Figure 2.**
*Trocar placement for Spiegel hernia.*

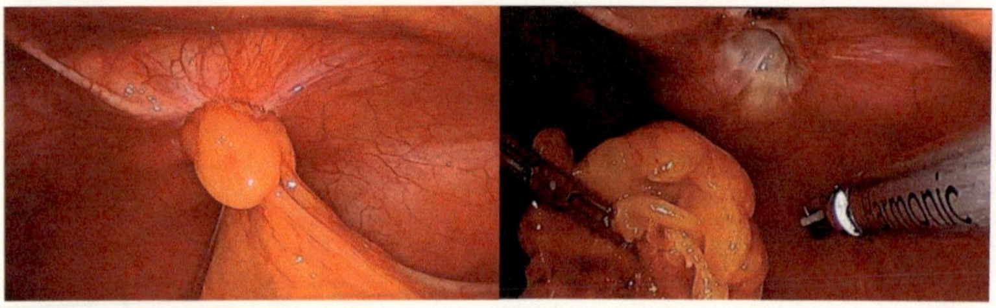

**Figure 3.**
*Transabdominal perspective to Spiegel hernia and reduction hernia component.*

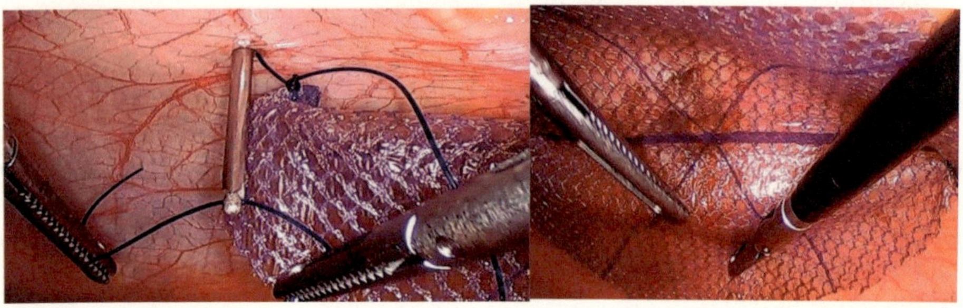

**Figure 4.**
*Suture catching and replacement of dual mesh.*

where the mesh will be hung from the upper and lower edges of the hernia defect, polypropylene sutures are caught one by one and pulled out of the abdomen; thus the mesh is fixed to the abdominal wall by its cranial and caudal ends. Mesh can be fixed to the abdominal wall by double-row stapling technique, with cyanoacrylate or with the help of various types of adhesives. When using staples, it is important to pay attention on neurovascular injuries to the abdominal wall.

Drains are not recommended in the abdomen, trocar is pulled under direct vision, and the abdomen is desufflated. The patient tolerated oral feeding on the same day of the surgery and discharged the on the next day (**Figure 4**).

## 2. Morgagni hernia

### 2.1 Introduction

Diaphragmatic hernias are among the rare abdominal hernias. The diaphragm may be called the roof of the abdomen due to its localization. The diaphragm connects the natural foramen, including the aorta, esophagus, inferior vena cava, and abdominal and thoracic spaces. Congenital defects of the diaphragm include posteromedial hernia, anteromedial hernia, central tendon defect, and diaphragm eventration [19]. Anteromedial diaphragmatic hernias constitute 2–3% of diaphragmatic hernias [20]. Ninety-one percent of these hernias can be located on the right side of the sternum and 5% on the left side of the sternum [21]. Diaphragmatic hernias can be congenital or post-traumatic.

### 2.2 History

Anteromedial diaphragmatic hernias were first recognized by an Italian anatomist and pathologist, Giovanni Batista Morgagni, in 1769 during an autopsy and were described in an article by the author entitled "The Sets and Causes of Diseases, Investigated by Anatomy" [22]. Since then, the disease has been called with Morgagni's name. In the pathophysiology of the disease, it is thought to be that there is a fusion defect in the midline of the diaphragm in the embryological period. Only 5% of Morgagni hernias are treated in adulthood, because most of these cases become symptomatic and treated in childhood. In the literature, different surgical approaches to the treatment of Morgagni hernia have been described and are divided into two types as transthoracic (median sternotomy, thoracotomy, or thoracoscopic assisted) and transabdominal (laparotomy or laparoscopic) [23]. There is still no consensus as to which is the best technique. However, since Kuster and colleagues reported their first laparoscopic repair in 1992, minimally invasive techniques have become the gold standard for diaphragmatic hernia repair due to the low recurrence rates, short postoperative hospital stay, and near-perfect cosmetic results [24].

### 2.3 General information

#### *2.3.1 Physiopathology*

Diagnosis of Morgagni hernia may rarely be delayed until adolescence and adulthood. This may be due to the asymptomatic course in some patients or the presentation of minimal atypical respiratory symptoms. The diagnosis is made after these minimal symptoms, which are generally atypical in elderly patients, are aggravated due to chronic constipation, chronic cough, pregnancy, obesity, or trauma.

#### *2.3.2 Symptomatology and clinical presentation*

The content of hernia is frequently omentum and transverse colon. Rarely, the small intestines and stomach can also be detected within the hernia sac.

Because hernia defect grows over time and there is a possibility of strangulation or incarceration of the organs it contains, surgical treatment is indicated when Morgagni hernia is diagnosed [25].

### *2.3.3 Diagnosis*

The gold standard for diagnosis is multislice abdominal computed tomography [26]. Abdominal CT examination, besides providing advanced anatomical information, enables us to determine the size of the hernia defect and which organs are formed or the presence of strangulation or incarceration. All this information is very important for preoperative planning.

## 2.4 Surgical indication

In a study in which Young et al. evaluated the results of 43 patients retrospectively regarding the choice of surgical technique, laparoscopy, laparotomy, and thoracotomy were found to have similar complication and recurrence rates [27]. In this study, 23% of the patients were treated laparoscopically and have shorter hospital stay than other techniques which was evaluated as the advantage of laparoscopy. In the repair of hernia defect, primary closure or mesh repair is available. The primary closure method can be performed technically intracorporeal or transfacial extracorporeal. Nonabsorbable 00 sutures are preferred for primary repair. In the transfacial extracorporeal technique, Endo Close® is inserted into the abdomen through mini incisions (described by Yamamato) [28], and the sutures that were previously sent into the abdomen are held one by one and pulled out of the abdomen and ligated to the hernia defect. The sutures are passed one by one 1 or 2 cm apart and are thrown to cover the cranial and caudal borders of the hernia defect. When sutures are hung outside the abdomen at the same time, it is seen that the hernia defect is closed. Square patches made of prolene mesh can be placed between the sutures so that the sutures do not interrupt the peritoneum and diaphragm.

### *2.4.1 Operating room*

The patient is taken to the operating table in the supine position with his legs open. 45° reverse Trendelenburg position is given. The laparoscopic tower is placed on the patient's right or left bedside (**Figure 5**).

### *2.4.2 Surgical instruments*

- Standard laparoscopy equipment consisting of camera, monitor, light, and insufflator (**Figure 6**).

- 10 mm diameter and 30° angle camera.

- Three trocar, one 10 mm, two 5 mm in diameter.

- Veress needle.

- Endo Instruments (Atraumatic clamp, dissector, scissors, hook, portegue, aspirator).

- Endo Close® sealing device with a diameter of –5 mm.

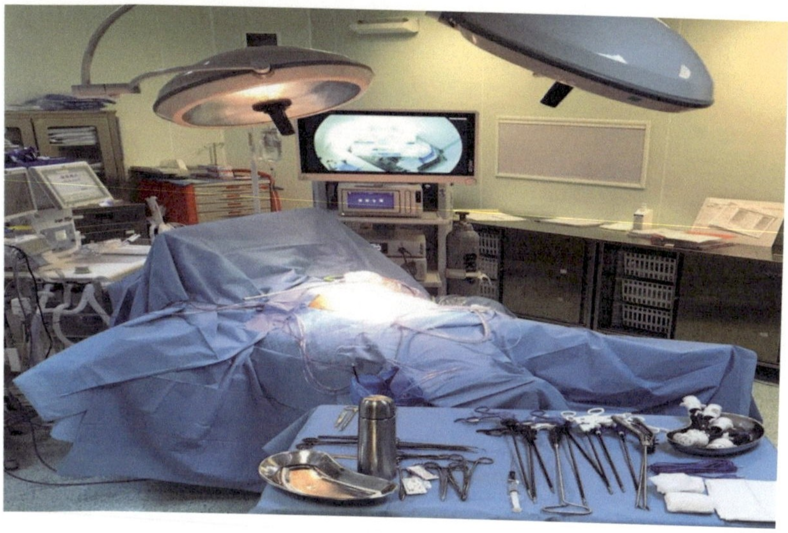

**Figure 5.**
*Operating room at a Morgagni hernia operation.*

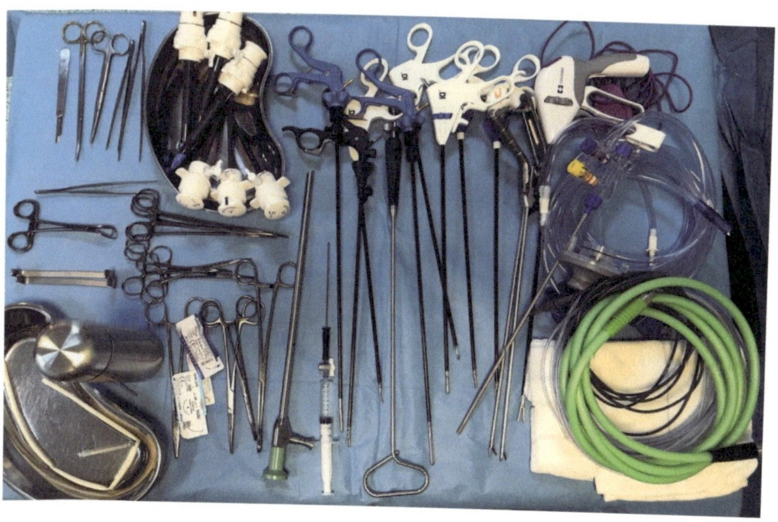

**Figure 6.**
*Conventional laparoscopic surgical instruments.*

- 20 x 30 cm composite or dual-coated special-shaped patch.
- Fixing material for mesh fixation and peritoneal closure (mechanical stapler, tissue glue, or nonabsorbable suture material).

### 2.4.3 Port placement and surgical technique

Under general anesthesia, the patient is stained and covered under sterile conditions, and entered into the abdomen with a left lateralized incision at a distance of 5 cm to umbilicus with the Hasson technique. After placing a 10 mm trocar and exploring the abdomen, one more 10 mm trocar and one more 5 mm trocars are inserted through the left and right midclavicular line under direct vision (**Figure** 7).

After exploration of the abdomen and the presence of concomitant hiatal hernia, the size of the hernia defect, its localization, and the organs it contains are

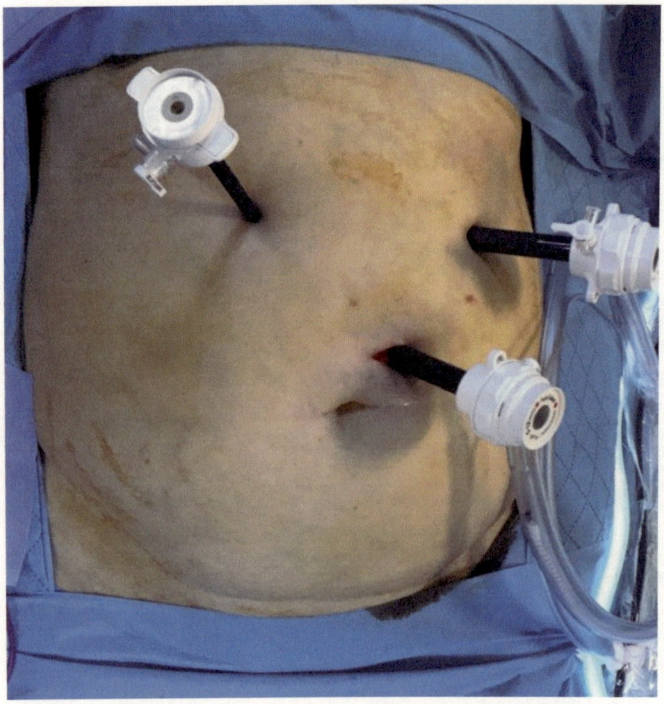

**Figure 7.**
*Trocar placement for Morgagni hernia.*

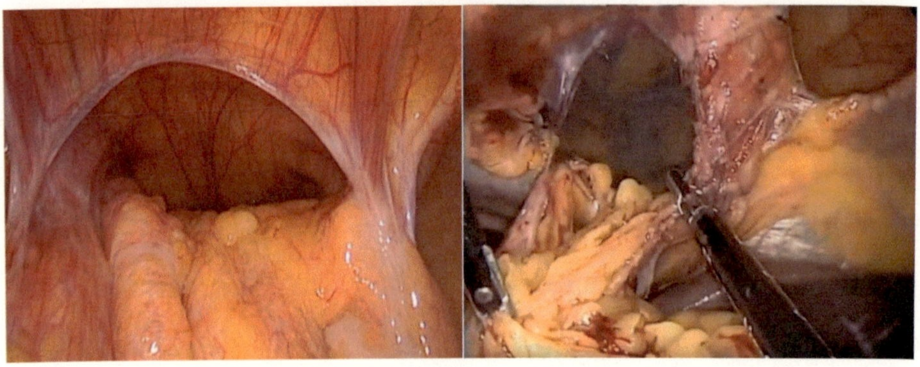

**Figure 8.**
*A huge right-sided Morgagni hernia and reduction of hernia.*

evaluated. After the reduction of the hernia contents to the abdomen, defect repair is started (**Figure 8**). As shown by Kuster et al., hernia sac dissection is not recommended due to the possible complications such as pneumothorax, hemothorax, and pulmonary effusion [29].

The primary repair option can be applied intracorporeally or extracorporeally. In the intracorporeal technique, the suture is applied superficially through the tendons and fibers of the diaphragm, with nonabsorbable suture material and with a separate technique, to cover the entire defect. In the extracorporeal technique, the sutures are applied by tying the nonabsorbable sutures that have been introduced trough the abdomen with the help of Endo Close® by pulling them out of the abdomen through millimeter incisions from the abdominal wall (**Figure 9**).

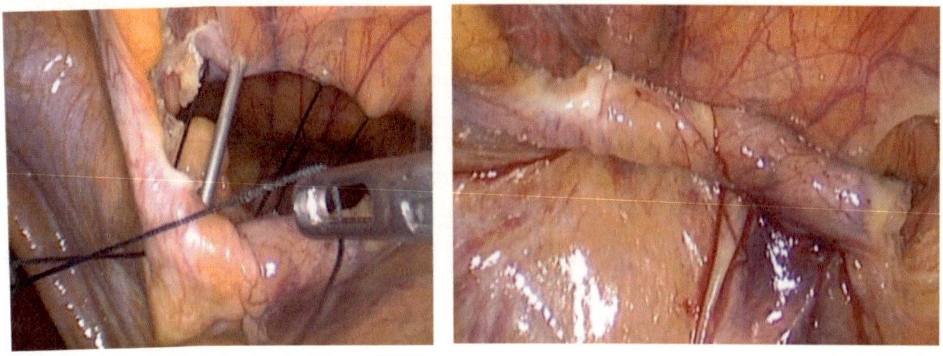

**Figure 9.**
*Intracorporeal suture technique using suture catcher.*

Both techniques should ensure that the defect is completely covered. Recurrence was not reported in patients who underwent thoracotomy and laparotomy including 36 cases performed by Aghajanzadeh et al. [30].

### 2.4.4 Use of mesh

Although the use of mesh is a standard practice in the repair of many hernias, the choice of mesh usage in Morgagni hernia may vary. Postoperative fistula development and migration to intrathoracic or intraabdominal cavity limit the use of composite mesh. However, it is recommended to use mesh in cases where the defect cannot be closed with primary suture technique due to the weak diaphragm or large defect (20–30 cm) [31–33]. In addition, Abraham et al. performed a series of 20 diseases in 6 patients with mesh repair and 4 patients with both mesh and primary repair, and no recurrence was reported at 20-month follow-up [34]. Similarly, in a series of three cases by Godazandeh et al., a polyvinylidene fluoride-coated patch was used, and no recurrence was reported at 18 months of follow-up [35]. Another option to consider when mesh repair is preferred is fixation of the mesh. It should be kept in mind that lung, heart, and diaphragmatic

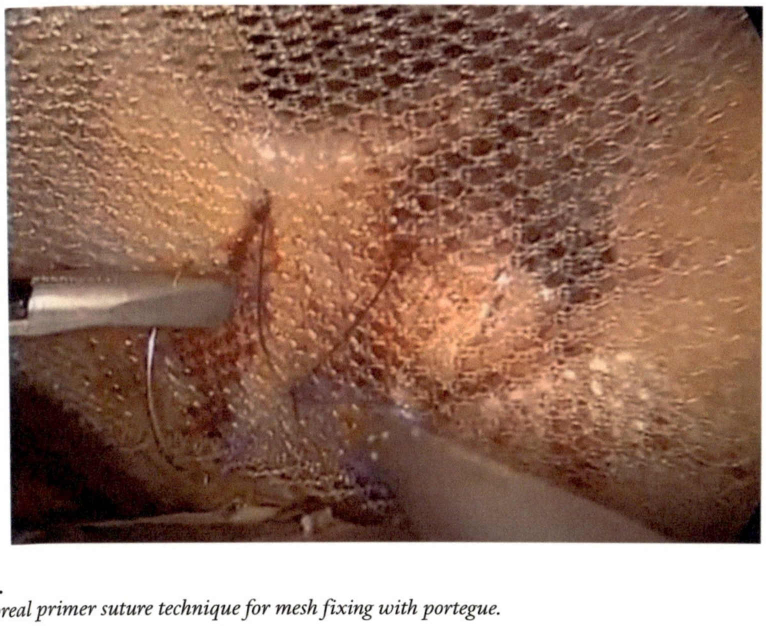

**Figure 10.**
*Intracorporeal primer suture technique for mesh fixing with portegue.*

injuries secondary to possible intrathoracic adhesions can be caused during fixation (Köckerling et al.). Köckerling et al. emphasized that the use of tacker should be avoided in mesh fixation as it can cause fatal complications [36]. When the pneumoperitoneum is evacuated, it is suggested that the fixation may not be applied with the help of the volume effect of the liver, but if it will be applied, it is recommended to fix the diaphragm with superficial sutures by intracorporeal or extracorporeal technique (**Figure 10**).

## Conflict of interest

The authors declare no conflict of interest.


## Author details

Emrah Akin[1], Baris Mantoglu[1], Fatih Altintoprak[2*] and Necattin Firat[1]

1 Department of General Surgery, Sakarya Research and Educational Hospital, Adapazari, Sakarya, Turkey

2 Faculty of Medicine, Department of General Surgery, Sakarya University, Adapazari, Sakarya, Turkey

*Address all correspondence to: fatihaltintoprak@yahoo.com

## References

[1] Mittal T, Kumar V, Khuller R, et al. Diagnosis and management of Spigelian hernia: A review of the literature and our experience. Journal of Minimal Access Surgery. 2008;**4**:95-98

[2] Spangen L. Spigelian hernia. World Journal of Surgery. 1989;**13**:573-580

[3] Skandalakis PN, Zoras O, Skandalakis JE, et al. Spigelian hernia: Surgical anatomy, embryology, and technique of repair. The American Surgeon. 2006;**72**:42-48

[4] Ruiz de la Hermosa A, Amunategui Prats I, Machado Liendo P, Nevarez Noboa F, Muñoz Calero A. Spigelian hernia. Personal experience and review of the literature. Revista Española de Enfermedades Digestivas. 2010;**102**:583-586

[5] Takayama S, Imafuji H, Funahashi H, Takeyama H. Laparoscopic Spigelian and inguinal hernia repair with the Kugel patch. Surgical Laparoscopy, Endoscopy and Percutaneous Techniques. 2010;**20**:e76-e78

[6] Carter JE, Mizes C. Laparoscopic diagnosis and repair of Spigelian hernia: Report of a case and technique. American Journal of Obstetrics and Gynecology. 1992;**167**:77-78

[7] Moreno-Egea A, Carrasco L, Girela E, Martín JG, Aguayo JL, Canteras M. Open vs laparoscopic repair of Spigelian hernia: A prospective randomized trial. Archives of Surgery. 2002;**137**:1266-1268

[8] Skandalakis PN, Zoras O, Skandalakis JE, Mirilas P. Spigelian hernia: Surgical anatomy, embryology, and technique of repair. The American Surgeon. 2006;**72**:42-48

[9] Read RC. Observations on the etiology of Spigelian hernia. Annals of Surgery. 1960;**152**:1004-1009

[10] Jones BC, Hutson JM. The syndrome of Spigelian hernia and cryptorchidism: A review of the paediatric literature. Journal of Paediatric Surgery. 2015;**50**:325-330

[11] Zimmerman LM, Anson BJ, Morgan EH, McVay CB. Ventral hernia due to normal banding of the abdominal muscles. Surgery. 1944;**78**:535

[12] Law TT, Ng KK, Ng L, et al. Elective laparoscopic totally extraperitoneal repair for Spigelian hernia: A case series of four patients. Asian Journal of Endoscopic Surgery. 2018;**11**(3):244-247. DOI: 10.1111/ases.12454

[13] River LP. Spigelian hernia. The Annals of Surgery. 1942;**116**:405

[14] Zimmerman LM, Anson BJ, Morgan EH, McVay CB. Ventral Hernia due to normal banding of the abdominal muscles. Surgical Gynaecology of Obstetric. 1944;**78**:535

[15] Webber V, Low C, Skipworth RJE, et al. Contemporary thoughts on the management of Spigelian hernia. Hernia. 2017;**21**(3):355-361. DOI: 10.1007/s10029-017

[16] Larson DW, Farley DR. Spigelian hernia: Repair and out- come for 81 patients. World Journal of Surgery. 2002;**26**:1277-1281

[17] Rankin A, Kostusiak M, Sokker A. Spiegelian hernia: Case series and review of the literatüre. Visceral Medicine. 2019;**35**(2):133-136. DOI: 10.1159/000494280

[18] Kelly ME, Courtney D, McDermott FD, Heeney A, Maguire D, Geoghegan JG, et al. Laparoscopic Spigelian hernia repair: A series of 40 patients. Surgical Laparoscopy, Endoscopy and Percutaneous Techniques. 2015;**25**:e86-e89

[19] Soldo I, Baca I, Sever M, et al. Laparoscopic treatment of Morgagni hernia: Report of three cases. Acta Clinica Croatica. 2017;**56**:318-322. DOI: 10.20471/acc.2017.56.0216

[20] Harrington SW. Clinical manifestations and surgical treatment of congenital types of diaphragmatic hernia. The Review of Gastroenterology. 1951;**18**(4):243-256

[21] Horton JD, Haffmann LJ, Hetz SP, et al. Presentation and management of Morgagni hernias in adults: A review of 298 cases. Surgical Endoscopy. 2008;**22**:1413-1420. DOI: 10.1007/s00464-008-9754-x

[22] Morgagni GB. The Seats and Causes of Diseases Investigated by Anatomy. Vol. 3. London, England: Millar & Caddell; 1769. p. 205

[23] Hassan A, Alabdrabalmaer M, Alealiuri M, et al. İncidental Morgagni hernia found during laparoscopic repair of hiatal hernia: Case report and review of literature. International Journal of Surgery Case Reports. 2019;**57**:97-101

[24] Kuster GG, Kline LE, Garzo G. Diaphragmatic hernia through the foramen of Morgagni: Laparosopic repair case report. Journal of Laparoendoscopic Surgery. 1992;**2**:93-100

[25] Comer JP, Clagett OT. Surgical treatment of hernia of the foramen of Morgagni. The Journal of Thoracic and Cardiovascular Surgery. 1966;**52**:461-468

[26] Li S, Liu X, Shen Y, et al. Laparoscopic repair of Morgagni hernia by artificial precardium patch in an adult obese patient. Journal of Thoracic Disease. 2015;7:754-757

[27] Young CM, Saddoughi SA, Aho JM, et al. Comparision of laparoscopic versus open surgical management of Morgagni hernia. The Annals of Thoracic Surgery. 2019;**107**(1):257-261

[28] Yamamato Y, Tanabe K, Hotta R, et al. Laparoscopic extra-abdominal suturing technique for the repair of Larrey's diaphragmatic hernia using the port closure needle (Endo Close®): A case report. International Journal of Surgery Case Reports. 2016;**28**:34-37

[29] Kuster GG, Kline LE, Garzo G. Diaphragmatic hernia through the foramen Morgagni: Laparoscopic repair case report. Journal of Laparoendoscopic Surgery. 1992;**2**:93-100

[30] Aghajanzadeh M, Khadem S, Khajeh JS, et al. Clinical presentation and operative repair of Morgagni hernia. Interactive CardioVascular and Thoracic Surgery. 2012;**15**(4):608-611. DOI: 10.1093/icuts/iu5203

[31] Mariceu D, Loubani M, O'Grady H. Late presentation of a large Morgagni hernia in an adult. BMJ Case Reports. 2014;**2014**. DOI: 10.1136/bcr.2013-202440

[32] Schiergens JS, Koch JG, Khalil PN, et al. Rigt-sided diaphragmatic rupture after repair of a large Morgagni hernia. Hernia. 2015;**19**(4):671-675. PMID: 26405726

[33] Huston JM, King H, Maresh A, et al. Hernia of Morgagni: A case report. The Journal of Thoracic and Cardiovascular Surgery. 2008;**135**(1):212-213. DOI: 10.1016/j.jtcus.2007.09.040

[34] Abraham V, Myla Y, Verghene S, et al. Morgagni-Larrey hernia. A review of 20 cases. The Indian Journal of Surgery. 2012;**74**(5):391-395. DOI: 10.1007/s12262-012-0431-x

[35] Godazandeh G, Mokhtari-Eshieve F. Laparoscopic repair

of Morgagni hernia:Three case presentation and the literatüre. Case Reports in Surgery. 2016;**2016**:42268539. DOI: 10.1155/2016/4268539

[36] Köckerling F, Schug-Pass C, Bittner R. A word of caution: Never use tacks for mesh fixation to the diaphragm! Surgical Endoscopy. 2018;**32**(7):3295-3302